Transform Your Core

Also by Mary El-Baz, Ph.D.

The Essence of Herbal and Floral Teas

Flavoring with Culinary Herbs: Tips, Recipes, and Cultivation

Easy and Healthful Mediterranean Cooking

Building a Healthy Lifestyle: A Simple Nutrition and Fitness Approach

Transform Your Core

6-Week Workbook

Mary El-Baz, Ph.D.

iUniverse, Inc.
New York Lincoln Shanghai

Transform Your Core
6-Week Workbook

iUniverse books may be ordered through booksellers or by contacting:

iUniverse
2021 Pine Lake Road, Suite 100
Lincoln, NE 68512
www.iuniverse.com
1-800-Authors (1-800-288-4677)

ISBN-13: 978-0-595-41697-4 (pbk)
ISBN-13: 978-0-595-86041-8 (ebk)
ISBN-10: 0-595-41697-7 (pbk)
ISBN-10: 0-595-86041-9 (ebk)

Printed in the United States of America

—To my wonderful sons and many friends who requested this simple plan as a shortcut in helping them deflate their 'spare tire'

Contents

Introduction

By a chance glance in the mirror one day, you discovered that your once drum-tight, sculpted midsection has been replaced by loose, apple-shaped belly flab, a spare tire. While you were busy with life, a few extra pounds crept up on you and settled right where your waist used to be. So now, you want to do something about it. You want to turn that flabby midsection back into its former firm and taut shape. The *Transform Your Core 6-Week Workbook* can help you do just that, by guiding you through a plan to turn your flabby, shapeless waistline into a slimmer and more defined one. In this six-week weight loss and fitness program, you will use this workbook to help you evaluate your weight (it's not just the numbers on your weight scale!), determine the right number of calories for you to maintain your weight, how blood sugar and stress influence weight gain and steps to control those, find out about foods that help stimulate weight loss, follow an eating plan for weight loss and build an eating plan for weight maintenance after the loss, tips on the importance of portion control, tips on eating away from home, and ways to improve your body fitness, including key fitness exercises that firm and strengthen your abdominal muscles during and after your weight loss. There are worksheets to chart and track your fitness program throughout the six weeks.

The *Transform Your Core* approach is to turn that flab into muscle, our bodies own fat-burning mechanism. Muscle speeds up fat burning; it is "metabolically active" and burns more calories than other body tissue even when you're not moving. Studies have estimated that for each pound of muscle that you add to your body, you burn an additional 35 to 50 calories per day. So, an extra 10 pounds of muscle will burn approximately 350 to 500 calories a day or an extra pound of fat every 7 to 10 days, without making any other changes. Isn't that sweet? When you combine exercise with the foods that fill you up, provide balanced nutrients, and promote muscle growth, you'll turn your fat into muscle.

What can you expect from the six-week *Transform Your Core* plan? In the first one to two weeks, you'll see a significant weight loss around your belly as your body adjusts to a change in eating, as you'll be gaining muscle mass and losing fat. You don't need to exercise during these first two weeks, but moderate walking can speed up the loss. A 5 to 8 pound loss is about the average weight loss during this period, depending on your own unique body build, frame size, age, and metabolism.

In the third and fourth weeks, you'll start moderating your eating plan to mainstream it into a daily eating plan for your lifestyle. You'll also start moderate strength and interval training to rev up your metabolism. Since, you've revved up your body's fat burning and muscle building metabolism, you'll feel the change in your body, as well as see some significant changes in your body shape. A 5 to 8 pound loss is about the average weight loss during this period, depending on your own unique body build, frame size, age, and metabolism.

In the fifth and sixth weeks, you'll be on your new lifestyle eating plan created by you! The previous two weeks of exercise will have geared up your body in using body fat for fuel in order to build muscle mass. Your upper body will be more toned, your waist smaller, and your abdominals starting to have definition again. By adding in exercises that specifically target your abdominal core muscles, you'll start fine-tuning the strength and enhance the definition of your core. From this point on, you'll be losing weight at a slower pace, working towards weight control rather than loss.

Enough already, now, let's transform your core!

Chapter 1

Evaluate Your Weight

There are a few key items in weight loss success which include the evaluation of your current weight, calorie consumption, types of foods you eat and their affect on your energy levels, and your stress levels and their affect on your weight. A common method of weight evaluation for adults is the body mass index (BMI). The BMI is a number that relates height to weight. However, your waist circumference measures abdominal fat. Both of these measures are used as indicators in assessing your overall health and any weight-related diseases and conditions.

An unbalanced diet can affect your body's delicate blood sugar and insulin metabolism balance which can affect your weight. For example, eating a chocolate candy bar increases the amount of sugar in the blood. When this occurs, the body releases the hormone insulin which causes sugar to be stored away and blood sugar levels to be lowered, which can trigger cravings for more sweets in order to stabilize blood sugar balance, which may leading to overeating and weight gain.

Stress can also affect your midsection weight in that the body uses the adrenal hormone cortisol to help balance your stress reactions. This hormone also plays a part in normalizing your blood sugar. When a stressor occurs, cortisol increases the blood sugar level in your body in a finely-tuned balance, but if stress becomes chronic then it can no longer maintain the balance. And that imbalance may lead to weight gain.

Let's explore all these a bit more.

BMI and Waist Circumference

The government developed a simple guideline called the Body Mass Index (BMI). The Body Mass Index (BMI) is an important tool to evaluate your weight and determine your risk of developing additional health problems. BMI is a common measure used to determine if you are overweight, obese, underweight, or normal. BMI takes into account a person's weight and height to gauge total body fat in adults. The higher the BMI is, the greater the risk of developing additional health problems. BMI *correlates* with body fat. The relationship between fatness and BMI differs with age and gender. For example, women are more likely to have a higher percentage of body fat than men for the same BMI. On average, older people may have more body fat than younger adults with the same BMI.

BMI equals a person's weight divided by height squared (BMI=kg/m^2 or lb/ft^2). It will, however, overestimate fatness in people who are muscular or athletic. Since BMI calculations use total body weight and not estimates of lean muscle mass and fat, it cannot determine between the overweight and the more muscular. BMI testing does not work for anyone under 18, for bodybuilders, or for pregnant or nursing women.

Women tend to believe they look their best at values between the range of 20 to 22 and men are usually satisfied with a BMI of 23 to 25. Generally, if your BMI falls within the range of 20 to 24.99, you are within the healthy weight range for your height and the risk of weight-related health problems is very small. Even though, a BMI under 20 may seem desirable, you may be at risk of underweight-related illness, such as disappearance of periods (women), bone loss, malnutrition, and other conditions.

If your BMI is 26 or more, your risk of health problems becomes higher. In a recent study, an increased rate of high blood pressure, diabetes, and heart disease was recorded at 27.3 for women and 27.8 for men. For any BMI 30 and over, you are considered obese. Experts agree that the "ideal" BMI scores should range from 19 to 25. Overweight is considered 25 to 29.9, and over 30 is obese. A person five-foot-nine and weighing 180 pounds has a BMI of 26.5, while at six-foot-one with the same weight the BMI would be 23.7.

Physicians rate obesity in various classes with associated weight-related health problems. It is a good idea to schedule a visit with your doctor to discuss your overall health condition and find out the best way to reduce your weight and risk.

BMI Is Not the Only Indicator of Health Risk

BMI is just one of many factors related to developing a chronic disease (such as heart disease, cancer, or diabetes). Other factors that may be important to look at when assessing your risk for chronic disease include diet, physical activity, waist circumference, blood pressure, blood sugar level, cholesterol level, and family history of disease.

Measure Your Waist Circumference

Another tool used to evaluate weight is your waist circumference. This is an especially helpful tool for people who are classified as overweight based on their BMI. That extra bit of fat, your spare tire, around the waist, is also a predictor of health problems. Having the information about waist circumference coupled with BMI gives extra insight into how serious a health problem overweight really poses. It is better to be pear-shaped rather than to have an apple-shaped silhouette. This is true even if your BMI shows you at a healthy weight. People with a pear-shaped body have hips wider than their shoulders because their bodies store fat there and on the thighs; women typically have a pear-shaped body. People with pear-shaped bodies carry their extra weight below the waistline, and do not seem to have as high a risk of developing health problems like diabetes, heart disease, stroke, or high blood pressure, than people with an apple-shaped body.

The apple-shaped body (body fat is stored around the middle: your abdomen, chest, and surround internal organs, such as the heart) is linked with health problems such as coronary heart disease, diabetes, stroke, high blood pressure and gall bladder disease.

The shape is predominantly a male phenomenon; although women are more prone to develop an apple shape in mid-life, particularly after menopause. This is because the female hormones are present in much smaller amounts and so the shape tends to become more 'male.'

To obtain a proper measurement, stand up and place a tape measure firmly, but not pressing into the skin, around your waist, between the bottom of your ribs and the top of your hipbones (the iliac crest), making sure the tape is parallel to the floor. The more your waist measurement increases, the greater your health risks. If you are a woman whose waist measures more than 35 inches or a man whose waist measures more than 40 inches, you may be at greater risk for health problems including diabetes, high blood fats, high blood pressure, and heart disease. This is true even if your BMI shows you at a healthy weight.

Impact of Your Weight on Your Overall Health

Look at your overall health; decide what impact your weight has and what you should work on to improve your health. The BMI will give you a baseline of your level of body fat and how much you should weigh. It's not the rule; it's just a guideline. It's unhealthy to have anxiety over a less-than-perfect body image. Physical activity and good nutrition are key factors in leading a healthy lifestyle and reducing risk for disease. You are taking steps to improve your health and fitness just by reading this book and becoming informed about health and fitness issues. Remember, a healthy mental attitude is just as important as physical fitness.

Calculating Your Body Mass Index

The BMI chart is an easy way to understand your body fitness. To find your Body Mass Index using the Body Mass Index Chart:

1. Find your height in inches, in the left-hand column.
2. Look across the row for your weight in pounds.
3. Then look up your BMI in the top column.

For example, you are 60 inches tall, and your weight is 118 pounds. Then, your Body Mass Index is 23 (Normal weight). If you are 64 inches in height and your weight is 173 pounds. Then, your Body Mass Index is 30 (Obese).

You can also calculate your BMI yourself by using either of these formulas:

BMI = Weight (in pounds) × 704.5 divided by (Height [in inches] × Height [in inches])
BMI = Weight (in kilograms) divided by (Height [in meters] × Height [in meters])

- Divide your height in centimeters by 2.54 to convert it into inches.
  Multiply your weight in kilograms by 2.2 to convert it into pounds.

For example, you are 158 centimeters in height. The calculation is 158 divided by 2.54 centimeters equals 62 inches. Your weight is 77 kilograms. The calculation is 77 multiplied by 2.2 pounds equals 169 pounds. Then, your Body Mass Index is 31 (Obese).

Note: If you have a BMI of 25 to 30 and waist circumference of greater than 35 (for women) or 40 or more (for men) *and* one or more risk factors, *or* your BMI is greater than 30 and you have one or more risk factors, then it's a good idea for you to talk to your doctor to see if you are at an increased risk for disease and discuss if weight loss will help. Even a small weight loss (just 10% of your current weight) may help lower the risk of disease. A complete health assessment by a physician is the best way to decide the right steps for you.

Body Mass Index Chart																					
BMI	19	20	21	22	23	24	25	26	27	28	29	30	31	32	33	34	35	36	37	38	39	40
Height	Weight in Pounds																					
58"	91	96	100	105	110	115	119	124	129	134	138	143	148	153	158	162	167	172	177	181	186	191
59"	94	99	104	109	114	119	124	128	133	138	143	148	153	158	163	168	173	178	183	188	193	198
60"	97	102	107	112	118	123	128	133	138	143	148	153	158	163	168	174	179	184	189	194	199	204
61"	100	106	111	116	122	127	132	137	143	148	153	158	164	169	174	180	185	190	195	201	206	211
62"	104	109	115	120	126	131	136	142	147	153	158	164	169	175	181	186	191	196	202	207	213	218
63"	107	113	118	124	130	135	141	146	152	158	163	169	175	180	186	191	197	203	208	214	220	225
64"	110	116	122	128	134	140	145	151	157	163	169	174	180	186	192	197	204	209	215	221	227	232
65"	114	120	126	132	138	144	150	156	162	168	174	180	186	192	198	204	210	216	222	228	234	240
66"	118	124	130	136	142	148	155	161	167	173	179	186	192	198	204	210	216	223	229	235	241	247
67"	121	127	134	140	146	153	159	166	172	178	185	191	198	204	211	217	223	230	236	242	249	255
68"	125	131	138	144	151	158	164	171	177	184	190	197	203	210	216	223	230	236	243	249	256	262
69"	128	135	142	149	155	162	169	176	182	189	196	203	209	216	223	230	236	243	250	257	263	270
70"	132	139	146	153	160	167	174	181	188	195	202	209	216	222	229	236	243	250	257	264	271	278
71"	136	143	150	157	165	172	179	186	193	200	208	215	222	229	236	243	250	257	265	272	279	286
72"	140	147	154	162	169	177	184	191	199	206	213	221	228	235	242	250	258	265	272	279	287	294
73"	144	151	159	166	174	182	189	197	204	212	219	227	235	242	250	257	265	272	280	288	295	302
74"	148	155	163	171	179	186	194	202	210	218	225	233	241	249	256	264	272	280	287	295	303	311
75"	152	160	168	176	184	192	200	208	216	224	232	240	248	254	264	272	279	287	295	303	311	319
76"	156	164	172	180	189	197	205	213	221	230	238	246	254	263	271	279	287	295	304	312	320	328

Note: The shaded area highlights the "healthy weight" BMI zone.

Activity Level

What is your activity level? Do you have a sedentary, lightly active, moderately active, or active lifestyle? Sedentary means a lifestyle that includes only the light physical activity associated with typical day-to-day life. Examples of sedentary activity include watching television, surfing the Internet, or reading e-mails. Lightly active means a lifestyle that includes physical activity such as biking or walking 2 hours a week, in addition to the light physical activity associated with typical day-to-day life. Moderately active means a lifestyle that includes physical activity equivalent to walking about 1.5 to 3 miles per day at 3 to 4 miles per hour, in addition to the light physical activity associated with typical day-to-day life. Examples of moderate physical activity besides walking briskly include mowing the lawn, dancing, swimming, or bicycling on level terrain. Active means a lifestyle that includes physical activity equivalent to walking more than 3 miles per day at 3 to 4 miles per hour, in addition to the life physical activity associated with typical day-to-day life. Examples of vigorous physical activity include jogging, mowing the lawn with a nonmotorized push mower, chopping wood, participating in high-impact aerobic dancing, swimming continuous laps, or bicycling uphill.

My BMI and Waist Circumference

Height: _____

Weight: _____

Waist: _____

BMI: _____

Activity
Level: Sedentary   Light   Moderate   Active

Right Number of Calories for Your Body

To maintain weight, you must consume the same calories that you expend. To lose weight, you must expend more calories than you consume. Since 3,500 calories equal one pound of weight, to lose one pound of weight, you must eat 3,500 fewer calories than your body needs to maintain its weight or burn 3,500 more calories through physical activity. Staying active is a key factor in staying healthy, fit, and being able to eat the foods you love. Studies have shown that active thin people generally take in an average of 600 calories a day more than their overweight peers, driving home the point that the amount of food you eat is not the only factor in losing weight. These people are active and working off more calories every day through physical activity and exercise and the increase in metabolism that regular physical activity induces.

So the simplest way to change your diet in order to lose weight is to concentrate on first *adding* lots of good food, not so much eating less and less food. You may be able to eat *as much* food as you ever have and still lose weight—if you eat the *right* kind of food.

Briefly, the food you eat is made up of the macronutrients of protein, carbohydrates, and fats, and the various micronutrients that include vitamins and minerals. Currently, the Institute of Medicine of the National Academies (an organization that provides science-based advice on matters of biomedical science, medicine, and health to the nation) recommends that adults get 45 to 65 percent of their daily calories from carbohydrates, 20 to 35 percent from fat, and 10 to 35 percent from protein. A good calorie intake balance for weight control is 30 percent protein, 30 percent fat, and 40 percent carbohydrate. By swapping these protein and carbohydrate calorie percentages, 40 percent protein and 30 percent carbohydrates, you can rev up your fat burning metabolism. Then, return to the daily calorie intake balance of 30 percent protein, 30 percent fat, and 40 percent carbohydrates to maintain the desire weight.

Here's how to determine the number of calories you'll need daily. First, determine your ideal weight. For men, add together 106 pounds for the first 5 feet, and 6 pounds for each additional inch. For women, add together 100 pounds for the first 5 feet, and 5 pounds for each additional inch. If you have a large frame, add 10 percent; if a small frame, subtract 10 percent. Now, figure your weight in kilograms by dividing your weight by 2.2 pounds (one kilogram). Then figure your ideal caloric intake by multiplying your weight in kilograms by 24 (hours in the day). Next, adjust your calories according to your activity level by factoring in your exercise and working activity. If you are a basically sedentary person, give yourself an additional 20 percent calories. If your activity is light, give yourself 30 percent more calories. If your activity is moderate, give yourself 40 percent more calories, and if your activity is vigorous, give yourself 50 percent more calories.

Finally, figure your percentage of protein, carbohydrates, and fats. Use the final calorie total and divide it into the percentages of protein (40), fats (30), and carbohydrates (30) for weight loss or the percentages of protein (30), fats (30), and carbohydrates (40) for weight control.

My Ideal Daily Calorie Total

Example (truncate number after the decimal point):

190 pounds as ideal weight for 6 foot tall man (106 + (6 x 12 inches) = 178)
Kilograms: 80 (178/2.2 = 80)
Calories: 1,920 (80 x 24=1,920)
Light activity: 1,920 x 0.30 = 576 extra
            1,920 + 576 = 2,496 total calories.
Percent Protein: 998 (2,496 x 0.40 = 998)
Percent Carbohydrates: 748 (2,496 x 0.30 = 748)
Percent Fats: 748 (2,496 x 0.30 = 748)

Height: _____

Ideal Weight: _____

Kilograms: _____

Calories: _____

Activity
Level: Sedentary   Light   Moderate   Active
             0.20   0.30   0.40   0.50

Extra
Calories: _____

Total
Calories: _____

Percent   Protein   Fats   Carbohydrates
             _____   _____   _____

Protein
Calories: _____

Fat
Calories: _____

Carbohydrate
Calories: _____

Blood Sugar Imbalance Influences Weight Gain

The foods we eat fuel our bodies enabling our cells to perform their specialized functions. Protein is the major component of our muscles and bones. In order for health to be maintained, we need to consume some protein every day. About four ounces of some lean meat, chicken, or fish can provide adequate protein. Among the most healthful sources of protein are cold-water fish such as mackerel, herring, and salmon, which contain a high-content of omega-3 fat which is beneficial for cardiovascular health. There are also a wide variety of soy products that are excellent alternatives for animal protein.

The fat in our foods is not the enemy, it is essential to maintaining life. In fact, many hormones, including estrogen, progesterone, and testosterone, are derived from fats. The vital lining around many nerves, as well as the membranes of cells, are fatty substances. You want to increase the "good" fats (monounsaturated and polyunsaturated) and reduce the "bad" fats (saturated and trans-fat) in your diet.

Carbohydrates provide our bodies with energy, fiber, and the feeling of satiety that we expect from food. Bread, pasta, rice, vegetables, and fruit are all carbohydrates; however some are more beneficial nutrient-wise than others! Vegetables provide your body with a wide variety of vitamins and minerals essential for its proper functioning, as well as fiber to help keep the digestive tract in good working order. Fruits also provide your body with essential nutrients besides vitamins and minerals, such as antioxidants and flavonoids. Grains provide vitamins, minerals and energy.

Our bodies break down carbohydrates into glucose or blood sugar. The level of blood sugar in our blood is one mechanism that controls hunger. When your blood glucose level falls below normal, you feel hungry. When you eat, and as your food is digested, carbohydrates in the food are converted into glucose and enter your bloodstream. As your blood sugar rises, your pancreas secretes insulin to clean up the excess blood sugar. This process repeats as your blood glucose levels fall below normal.

The glycemic index (GI) is a numerical system of ranking carbohydrate foods according to how quickly they release glucose into your bloodstream. Foods that are at the higher end of the glycemic index break down quickly during digestion, causing rapid blood sugar changes that can affect your mood and desire to eat again. Foods that are on the lower end of the glycemic index usually break down more slowly, releasing glucose gradually into the bloodstream, thus maintaining a stable blood sugar level over a longer period. For example, if your blood sugar is low and continues to drop during your workout, you would prefer to eat a carbohydrate that would raise your blood sugar quickly. On the other hand, if you would like to keep your blood sugar from dropping during a few hours of mild activity, you may prefer to eat a carbohydrate that has a lower glycemic index and longer action time. A food's glycemic index is based on glucose, which is one of the fastest carbohydrates available. Glucose is given an arbitrary value of 100 and other carbohydrates are given a number relative to glucose. A GI of 70 or more is high, a GI of 56 to 69 inclusive is medium, and a GI of 55 or less is low. Faster carbohydrates (higher numbers) are great for raising low blood sugars and for covering brief periods of intense exercise. Slower carbohydrates (lower numbers) are helpful for preventing overnight drops in the blood sugar and for long periods of exercise.

High-glycemic foods can cause us to be hungrier more often, thus we overeat (ingesting more calories than our bodies can use), which leads to obesity. Here's what happens when you eat a high-glycemic food or meal. There is a rapid rise in your blood sugar level. This overstimulates the pancreas to release a much larger amount of insulin. This large amount of insulin rapidly cleans up the excess sugar in your bloodstream, causing the blood sugar level to dip quickly below normal. Now you're hungry again! So you eat once more after you have just eaten! This process can lead to overeating and weight gain. Eating low-glycemic foods helps slow down this cycle by delaying the return of hunger. As a result, meals are spaced further apart, increasing the satiety of foods eaten, sustaining more energy, maintaining stable blood sugar levels, and reducing calorie intake. This, ultimately, is weight control.

Low-glycemic eating plans focus on reducing the intake of foods that elevate insulin and stimulate fat storage. Non-carbohydrate foods, such as protein and fats, do not raise your blood sugar much, if at all. Low-glycemic foods can be mixed with modest quantities of high-glycemic foods without losing their hunger-reducing effect. Keeping the higher-glycemic foods to a minimum and eating them in combination with low-glycemic foods will not significantly elevate insulin levels. Just make sure that the foods you choose have a significant amount of soluble fiber! That is, fiber that slows digestion, which reduces the glycemic effect. Also, even though low-glycemic foods do not stimulate fat storage as efficiently as high-glycemic foods, they still contain calories. Serving and portion sizes do matter. The more carbohydrates you eat, the more insulin produced by the body, and the more fat storage that occurs.

The **Glycemic Index of Common Foods** table displays a table of the glycemic index for common foods which includes breads, cereals, grains, vegetables, fruits, dairy, and snacks. Please keep in mind that the impact a food will have on your blood sugar depends on many other factors such as ripeness, cooking time, fiber and fat content, time of day, blood insulin levels, and recent activity. You can use the glycemic index as a tool to improve your diet.

Glycemic Index of Common Foods

	Low Glycemic Foods		Moderately Glycemic Foods		Highly Glycemic Foods	
	Choose most often		Choose more often		Choose less often	
Breads						
	Pumpernickel	41	Pita	57	White bread	70
	Heavy mixed grain	49	Sourdough	57	Bagel, white	72
	100% stone ground whole wheat	60	Whole wheat	69	Rye, dark	76
	Apple cinnamon muffin	44	Hamburger bun	61	Baguette, French	95
	Oatmeal & raisin muffin	41	Blueberry muffin	59		
			Croissant	67		
Cereal						
	All-Bran®	42	Grape-Nuts®	67	Bran flakes	74
	Bran Buds w/ Psyllium™	45	Shredded wheat	67	Cheerios®	74
	Oatmeal (old-fashioned)	48	Life®	66	Rice Kripsies®	82
	Muesli, natural	54	Cream of wheat	66	Corn flakes	84
	Special K®	54			Corn Chex®	83
					Raisin bran	73
					Total®	76
Grains						
	Barley	25	Buckwheat (kasha)	54	Short-grain rice	70

	Low Glycemic Foods		Moderately Glycemic Foods		Highly Glycemic Foods	
	Choose most often		Choose more often		Choose less often	
Grains						
	Parboiled or converted rice	38	Basmati rice	58		
	Fettuccine	40	Couscous	65		
	Spaghetti	42	Brown rice	66		
	Macaroni	47	Wild rice	57		
	Bulgur	48	White rice	64		
	Linguine	52				
	Vermicelli	35				
Vegetables						
	Sweet potato	52	New white potato	59	Baking potato, Russet	85
	Yam	54	Sweet corn	56	French fries	75
	Lentils	30	Beets	64	Parsnips	97
	Chickpeas	34			Rutabaga	72
	Kidney beans	29			Mashed potatoes	70
	Split peas	32			Baked red potato	93
	Soy beans	18				
	Baked beans	48				
	Carrots	47				
	Green beans	30				
	Pinto beans	39				
	Navy beans	38				
Fruit						
	Pear	36	Pineapple	59	Watermelon	72
	Apple	38	Cantaloupe	65	Dried dates	103
	Apple juice	41	Raisins	64		
	Peach	42	Apricots	57		
	Grapefruit	25	Papaya	58		
	Grapefruit juice	48				

	Low Glycemic Foods		Moderately Glycemic Foods		Highly Glycemic Foods	
	Choose most often		Choose more often		Choose less often	
Fruit						
	Pineapple juice	46				
	Plum	39				
	Kiwi	47				
	Mango	55				
	Orange	44				
	Orange juice	57				
	Strawberries	40				
	Grapes	46				
	Banana	55				
	Cherries	22				
Dairy						
	Whole milk	27	Ice cream, full fat, vanilla	61		
	Skim milk	32				
	Low-fat yogurt, plain	14				
	Low-fat yogurt, fruit	33				
	Ice milk, vanilla	50				
Snacks	Peanuts	14	Popcorn	55	Soda crackers	72
	Chocolate bar	49	Stoned Wheat Thins®	67	Rice cakes	80
	Snickers® bar	41	Ryvita® rye crisps	60	Pretzels	83
	Strawberry jam	51	Mars bars	65	Graham crackers	74
	Honey	55	Oatmeal cookie	57	Vanilla wafers	80
			Potato chips	56	Corn chips	72
			PowerBar® bars	58		
			Wheat Thins®	67		

	Low Glycemic Foods		Moderately Glycemic Foods		Highly Glycemic Foods	
	Choose most often		Choose more often		Choose less often	
Other						
	Cheese tortellini	50	Black bean soup	64		
			Green pea soup	66		
			Mac n' cheese	64		
			Pizza, cheese & tomato	60		

Source: Adapted from Foster-Powell, K., Holt, S., Brand-Miller, J. (2002), International table of glycemic index and glycemic load values, *American Journal of Clinical Nutrition.* 76, 5-76

Stress Hormone (Cortisol) Influences Weight Gain

Cortisol is one of several hormones made in the adrenal glands. It is important for normal carbohydrate metabolism and response to stress. Cortisol is also known as the "stress hormone." The primary responsibility of cortisol is to activate the immune system; it also is involved with the metabolism of glucose and can cause elevation of the blood sugar level. Cortisol has many actions in the body, and one ultimate goal of cortisol secretion is to provide energy.

Cortisol stimulates fat and carbohydrate metabolism for fast energy, and stimulates insulin release and maintenance of blood sugar levels. The end result of these actions is an increase in appetite. Thus chronic stress, or poorly managed stress, may lead to cortisol levels that stimulate your appetite, with the end result being weight gain or difficulty losing unwanted pounds. Cortisol not only promotes weight gain, but it can also affect where you put on the weight. Studies have shown that stress and elevated cortisol tend to cause fat deposition in the abdominal area rather than in the hips. This fat deposition has been referred to as "toxic fat" since abdominal fat deposition is strongly correlated with the development of cardiovascular, disease including heart attacks and strokes.

Whether your stress levels will result in high cortisol levels and weight gain is not readily predictable. The amount of cortisol secreted in response to stress can vary among individuals, with some persons being innately more "reactive" to stressful events.

Experts agree that stress management is a critical part of weight loss regimens, particularly in those who have elevated cortisol levels. Exercise is the best and fastest method for weight loss in this case, since exercise leads to the release of endorphins, which have natural stress-fighting properties and can lower cortisol levels. Activities such as yoga and meditation can also help lower stress hormone levels. To effectively reduce elevated cortisol due to stress, lifestyle changes are essential.

Begin recognizing and managing your stress by:

- **Developing relaxation skills.** Several relaxation techniques are discussed later in this section.

- **Paying attention to physical health.** Stress results from a combination of physical and mental factors. If your body isn't able to handle these challenges, you aren't going to be capable of effectively managing your stress level.

- **Exercising regularly.** Exercise not only stimulates release of endorphins, the body's natural stress-fighters, but it also helps lower cortisol and other stress hormone levels.

- **Prioritizing commitments and responsibilities.** Learn to differentiate between mandatory obligations and commitments you've made due to guilt, to satisfy others, or to fulfill unrealistic expectations of yourself. Learning to say no can help you reduce the stress of excessive demands on your time and energy. If your stress is job-related, it is time to think about whether that job is worth the poor health, physical and mental. This may be your body's way to telling you to move on to a different job or line of work.

- **Getting more sleep.** Poor sleep and stressful days can evolve into a vicious cycle. The inability to sleep may actually make some of us more prone to stress. Doctors studies have shown that levels of cortisol were higher in people with chronic insomnia and suggested that people with insomnia might have a hyperactive body response to stress.

- **Reducing caffeine.** Caffeine raises the production of cortisol. Studies have shown that as little as two to three cups of coffee can raise your cortisol level. Heavy coffee consumption can lead to a state of adrenal gland exhaustion, where the adrenal glands are no longer able to respond adequately to stress by releasing enough adrenaline. Adrenal insufficiency can then lead to a host of other problems, including a weakened immune response, anxiety, and panic attacks. Caffeine also interferes with adenosine, a brain chemical that normally has a calming effect, and raises the level of lactate, a biochemical known to produce panic attacks. Switching to tea, therefore reducing your caffeine intake, can sometimes make all the difference.

Stress Reduction Techniques

While a certain amount of stress can be beneficial, stimulating the body and mind to improve your performance, too much stress causes over-stimulation and leads to physical and mental illnesses. Relaxation techniques, when used consistently, can prove effective in controlling stress by helping you reach a state of mental calm, even when you are in the middle of a stressful situation. Here are a few easy relaxation techniques you can practice to prevent or ease stress-induced illness.

The Relaxation Response

The Relaxation Response is a simple technique that can relieve stress and tension. It was developed by Herbert Benson, M.D., at Harvard Medical School. He conducted extensive testing and included the results in his book, *The Relaxation Response.*

- Select fifteen minutes in your day, preferably early evening, before dinner when you'll be free of distractions. If you prefer to relax later in the evening, do so two hours after any meal, since the digestive processes seem to interfere with the elicitation of the relaxation response. Keep a watch or clock nearby so you can check your time periodically.

- Choose a focus word or short phrase that has some resonance for you. No, it does not need to be "Ohm"; it could be "Serenity Now." Just pick a word or words that are calming to you.

- Sitting quietly in a comfortable position in a comfortable chair, and close your eyes. Breathe slowly and normally, repeating the word silently as you exhale.

- Consciously relax your muscles, beginning from your toes, moving up to your feet, then ankles, calves, knees, thighs, hips, stomach, chest, shoulders, upper arms, elbows, lower arms, wrists, hands, fingers, then your neck, and finally, your head.

- Keep breathing evenly and keep repeating your word or phrase. Sometimes, other thoughts will come whirling in like a hamster running in its exercise wheel. Acknowledge these thoughts, and let them move through you; you can address them after you finish.

- When fifteen minutes have elapsed, sit quietly for a few minutes with your eyes still closed, and then open them.

- You will most likely be in a more peaceful and a calmer state. This state is your body's natural relaxation response. See, easy, without any fancy mediation techniques to learn.

Breath Counting

Breath counting is another simple relaxation technique that takes ten minutes.

- Select ten minutes in your day when you'll be free of distractions. Keep a watch or clock nearby so you can check your time periodically.

- Sit quietly in a comfortable position in a comfortable chair, and close your eyes. Take a few deep breaths. Then breathe naturally. It should be quiet and slow.

- Count 1 to yourself as you exhale.

- Upon the next exhaled breath, count 2. Continue counting your exhaled breath up to 5.

- Begin a new cycle of counting five breaths. Sometimes, your mind will wander and you may find yourself counting more than five breaths. That's okay; just go back and start at 1 again.

- When ten minutes have elapsed, sit quietly for a few minutes with your eyes still closed, and then open them.

Visualization or Guided Imagery

In addition to reducing stress, visualization can direct the stress to create a more positive mental performance. Many athletes use visualization during training.

- Select ten minutes in your day when you'll be free of distractions. Keep a watch or clock nearby so you can check your time periodically.

- Sit quietly in a comfortable position in a comfortable chair, and close your eyes. Take a few deep breaths. Then breathe naturally. It should be quiet and slow.

- Imagine a relaxing scene. If you enjoy relaxing at the beach, imagine a beach scene. If you prefer a garden, then imagine a garden scene. Imagine all the details of the scene with vibrant colors, sounds, aromas, tastes, textures, and emotion. For example, if you find the beach a place of relaxation, perhaps you'd see the blue water and sky, white sand and caps of the waves, and green palm trees. You'd likely hear the waves, the seagulls, and the wind. You'd smell fish and taste the salt in the air. You'd feel the smoothness and the wetness of the water and the grittiness of the sand. You'd likely experience a sense of peace and serenity. The use of visualization can take you on a trip for little effort and without any expense.

- When your mind wanders, bring it firmly back to your scene. Concentrate on the image and make every effort to exclude everything else. This may be difficult at first, but will become easier with practice.

- When ten minutes have elapsed, sit quietly for a few minutes with your eyes still closed, and then open them.

Using Visualization for Stress at Work

If you know that you have a stressful meeting, a confrontation, or a social situation coming up, you can prepare yourself by using visualization.

- Select ten minutes when you'll be free of distractions. Keep a watch or clock nearby so you can check your time periodically.
- Sit quietly in a comfortable position in a comfortable chair, and close your eyes. Take a few deep breaths. Then breathe naturally. It should be quiet and slow.
- Imagine the meeting, confrontation, or social situation—the location, the people present, and agendas at hand.
- Rehearse the various scenes in your mind; picture what will produce the stress, however small the detail is.
- Distance yourself from the problem and relax, breathing deeply and evenly. At first, you may find that tension arises, but as you continue the tension will ease away.
- Once you have confronted and overcome one problem, go to the next one.
- When ten minutes have elapsed, sit quietly for a few minutes with your eyes still closed, and then open them.
- By the time the meeting, confrontation, or social situation occurs, you will have reduced the stress it would have caused to a very manageable level or to no stress at all.

Autogenic Training

This relaxation technique is similar to visualization in that it works through self-suggestion but focuses on specific muscle relaxation. It can be helpful in reducing nervous tension, such as performance anxiety before an exam. This technique is popular in Europe and has been gaining increased acceptance in the United States and in other countries.

- Select fifteen minutes when you'll be free of distractions. Keep a watch or clock nearby so you can check your time periodically.

- Sit quietly in a comfortable position in a comfortable chair, and close your eyes. Take a few deep breaths. Then breathe naturally. It should be quiet and slow.

- Basic training starts with six simple phrases that must be practiced repeatedly in sequence. At the advanced level, additional suggestions may be incorporated into the training program. The six phrases are as follows:

  o My body is very heavy (promotes muscle relaxation).

  o I am very warm (relaxes your blood vessels and enhances circulation).

  o My heartbeat is calm and regular (regulates your pulse).

  o My breathing is calm and regular (relaxes your lungs and airways).

  o My abdomen is warm and relaxed (relaxes your stomach and exercises the abdominal wall).

  o My forehead is cool and clear (relieves tension in your head).

- Repeat the phrases and before the end of your relaxation period, add in a phrase that relates to your ailment, such as "my head is cool and clear" if you have a headache.

- When fifteen minutes have elapsed, sit quietly for a few minutes with your eyes still closed, and then open them.

Passive Relaxation Through Therapeutic Massage

Being massaged is another method to combat the symptoms of stress. Massage therapists work directly on the muscles and ligaments of the body. The massage relieves muscle tension and improves circulation and lymph drainage, thus helping the body rid itself of toxins. Its effect on the nervous system to calm, soothe, and give an overall sense of well-being is an ideal relaxation technique for busy people. There are various massage techniques, including sports, deep tissue, neuromuscular, and Swedish.

Mindful Meditation

There are many types of meditation that you can practice to relax the mind and trigger the body's natural relaxation response. Many forms of meditation, such as Transcendental Meditation, require a teacher. However, mindfulness has been defined as the state of attention and awareness of present experiences, bringing yourself in touch with inner wisdom and to a moment-by-moment awareness of what you experience and feel. Paying attention to sounds, breathing rhythms, inner feelings, and your reaction patterns to specific situations are all part of being mindful. You can meditate mindfully by following these simple steps.

- Select fifteen minutes in your day when you'll be free of distractions. Keep a watch or clock nearby so you can check your time periodically.

- Sit quietly in a comfortable position in a comfortable chair, and close your eyes. Take a few deep breaths. Then breathe naturally. It should be quiet and slow.

- Gently notice your breathing. Refrain from trying to control or alter it in any way.

- Notice how your breath changes on its own accord. It may vary in speed, rhythm, or depth, and there may even be occasions when your breath seems to stop for a time. Whatever happens with your breathing, observe it without trying to cause any changes.

- Keep your focus on your breathing for the entire period.

- When fifteen minutes have elapsed, sit quietly for a few minutes with your eyes still closed, and then open them.

My Stressors

Identify 3 or 4 of your primary stressors:

1. _____
2. _____
3. _____
4. _____

Identify 3 or 4 stress reduction techniques you want to practice:

1. _____
2. _____
3. _____
4. _____

Chapter 2

Transform Your Core Plan

In this chapter, you'll discover foods that help stimulate weight loss and use them in an eating plan that jump starts your weight loss and also in an eating plan for weight maintenance after the loss. You'll also learn about the importance of portion control and how to select and enjoy healthy foods when you eat out. Additionally, you'll be changing your fitness activities to boost your health along with your weight loss.

Fat Loss Stimulating Foods

Berries: Strawberries, cranberries, blackberries, raspberries, and cherries are all low-glycemic fruit which besides providing vitamins and minerals, satisfy your sweet-tooth and maintain your blood sugar balance.

Nuts and Seeds: Nuts and seeds are rich in protein, fiber, vitamins, and minerals, as well as being highly concentrated in monounsaturated and polyunsaturated essential fatty acids (fats). Essential fatty acids are essential for stored energy. Nuts and seeds contain liberal amounts of omega-3 (primarily flaxseed) and omega-6 essential fatty acids which play an important part in the body in fighting cardiovascular disease, reducing cholesterol levels and inflammation, and relieving arthritis. Choose from among almonds, walnuts, pecans, Brazil nuts, hazel nuts, pine nuts, macadamia nuts, sesame seeds, flaxseeds, sunflower seeds, pumpkin seeds, peanuts, and nut butters. Ground flaxseeds have a wonderful nutty flavor and can be sprinkled into drink shakes and onto cereals and yogurt.

Whey Protein Powder: This supplemental form of protein will help maximize your retention of fat burning lean muscle tissue. Whey protein has a high bio-absorption level in the body, allowing muscles to remain structurally supported and metabolism in high gear.

Blender Shakes: Easily and quickly made with milk, yogurt, whey powder, nut butter, fiber-rich oatmeal and bran, or fruit, blender shakes are satisfying and filling, sustaining you from one meal to the next without a precipitous drop in energy. Commercially-prepared meal replacement shakes can also be used as a quick substitute.

Multivitamin and Mineral Supplement: Subtle vitamin deficiencies can result from excessive consumption of nutrient-depleted foods such as refined sugar and white flour, from inadequate intake of vitamin-rich fruits and vegetables, and from nutrient losses due to processing, prolonged heating, or storage of foods. Sometimes you won't be eating whole, unprocessed foods that contain a wide array of beneficial substances besides vitamins, such as carotenoids, flavonoids, and natural antioxidants. You'll be eating at restaurants and fast-food chains. Remember, vitamin supplementation is not an adequate substitute for a good diet. The best approach to disease prevention and weight control is to eat properly and to take a multivitamin.

Green Tea: This supplement has all the benefits of a stimulant in enhancing metabolism. The caffeine in green tea increases metabolism, caloric burning, and weight loss, without negatively affecting the body.

Rev Up Plan

Follow this eating plan for the first two weeks of your transformation. A seven day meal plan is presented and you can modify it with some of the listed alternative meals and also substitute similar food items for those listed, for example walnuts for almonds, an orange for an apple, a piece of string cheese instead of a slice of cheese.

Here are important points of the plan:

- Drink at least eight 8-ounce glasses of water throughout the day, plain or sparkling with a lemon or lime slice
- Eat every 3 hours to maintain your energy level

- Unless specified, eat moderately-sized food portions, don't fill a 12-inch plate to the edges with food
- Recipes follow the daily menus for the items marked with an asterisk (*)
- No need to count calories during these two weeks
- Cut down or avoid alcoholic drinks altogether, these add excess and empty calories that you don't need just now
- Practice stress reduction techniques
- No exercise required, but you can add a daily light to moderate walking fitness activity to speed up weight loss
- Chart your progress every week on the fitness charts found in Chapter 4

Day 1

Breakfast
8- to 12-ounce Quick Blender Shake* or commercial meal-replacement shake

Snack
2 teaspoons peanut butter or other nut butter (almond, cashew) and unlimited amount of raw veggies (carrots, celery, broccoli, cauliflower, cherry tomatoes)

Lunch
Roast beef sandwich on whole-grain bread with lettuce, tomato, mustard or low-fat mayo; 1 cup 1% or fat-free milk or 1 cup iced or hot green tea; and 1 medium apple

Snack
1 ounce almonds and 1½ cup berries (strawberries, raspberries, blueberries, or blackberries)

Dinner
Meatball sandwich on whole-grain Kaiser roll with reduced-fat mozzarella cheese

Snack
8- to 12-ounce Quick Blender Shake* or commercial meal-replacement shake

Day 2

Breakfast
Egg and lean ham sandwich on whole-grain English muffin

Snack
2 teaspoons peanut butter or other nut butter and 1 bowl oatmeal or high-fiber cereal (All-Bran® or Fiber One®)

Lunch
Chef salad made with leafy lettuce, hard-boiled egg, black or green olives, low-fat cheddar cheese, tomatoes, shredded carrots, red cabbage, and sprinkled with grated Parmesan cheese

Snack
3 slices deli turkey and 1 large apple or pear

Dinner
Grilled or sautéed chicken breast served with commercially or home prepared salsa

Snack
1 ounce almonds and ½ cup cubed cantaloupe

Day 3

Breakfast
8- to 12-ounce Quick Blender Shake* or commercial meal-replacement shake

Snack
1 ounce almonds and 1 ounce raisins

Lunch
Tuna-egg salad made with low-fat mayo on whole-grain Kaiser sandwich roll

Snack
2 sticks string cheese and unlimited amount of raw veggies

Dinner
Grilled or sautéed marinated lean steak (such as London Broil or flank steak)

Snack
8- to 12-ounce Quick Blender Shake* or commercial meal-replacement shake

Day 4

Breakfast
1 slice whole-grain bread with 1 teaspoon peanut butter, 1 cup All-Bran® or Fiber One® cereal with 1 cup 1% or fat-free milk and 1½ cup berries

Snack
6-ounce container of plain or vanilla low-fat yogurt and 11.5-ounce can of low-sodium vegetable juice

Lunch
Turkey bacon, lettuce, and tomato sandwich on whole-wheat bread

Snack
3 slices deli roast beef and ½ cup canned tangerine segments, drained

Dinner
Roast beef, grilled onions, and peppers with reduced-fat cheddar cheese on a whole-grain French sandwich roll

Snack
2 teaspoons peanut butter or other nut butter (almond, cashew) and 1 cup low-fat ice cream

Day 5

Breakfast
8- to 12-ounce Quick Blender Shake* or commercial meal-replacement shake

Snack
1 ounce almonds and ½ cup sliced kiwi

Lunch
Salmon-egg salad made with low-fat mayo on a whole-grain French sandwich roll

Snack
3 slices deli roast beef and 1 large pear

Dinner
Chicken or turkey chili served over brown rice

Snack
8- to 12-ounce Quick Blender Shake* or commercial meal-replacement shake

Day 6

Breakfast
8- to 12-ounce Quick Blender Shake* or commercial meal-replacement shake

Snack
1 bowl high-fiber cereal and 6-ounce container plain or vanilla low-fat yogurt

Lunch
Leftover chicken or turkey chili served over brown rice

Snack
2 teaspoons peanut butter or other nut butter (almond, cashew) spread on 1 or 2 slices whole-grain bread

Dinner
Free meal—have whatever you like: a hamburger and fries, taco, burrito, shrimp pasta, chicken wings, grilled sausage, grilled or breaded chicken fingers and ranch dipping sauce, meat and mashed potatoes, steak and baked potato with your favorite toppings, etc.

Snack
8- to 12-ounce Quick Blender Shake* or commercial meal-replacement shake

Day 7

Breakfast
Egg and lean ham sandwich on whole-grain English muffin

Snack
2 teaspoons peanut butter or other nut butter and 11.5-ounce can low-sodium vegetable juice

Lunch
2 scrambled eggs, 2 slices whole-grain toast, 1 banana, and 1 cup 1% or fat-free milk or hot green tea

Snack
3 slices deli roast beef and 1 slice fat-free cheese

Dinner
Chili Hot Beans with turkey kielbasa

Snack
1 ounce almonds or walnuts and 1 cup low-fat ice cream

Lunch and Snack Alternatives

Lunch

- ½ whole-wheat bagel, toasted, topped with 1 tablespoon peanut butter or other nut butter and 1 canned pineapple ring, and 1 cup of calcium-fortified grapefruit juice
- 1 whole-wheat pita bread filled with ⅓ cup canned, drained beans (kidney, garbanzo, or black), or ⅓ cup hummus, 1 ounce low-fat cheddar cheese, and 1 teaspoon chopped red onion; 2 plums or 1 nectarine; and 1 cup of low-fat milk or green tea

Snacks

- ¾ cup low-fat ice cream and 1½ cup berries
- 1½ slices fat-free cheese and 11.5-ounce can low-sodium vegetable juice
- 3 slices low-sodium deli turkey breast and 1 or 2 slices whole-grain bread
- 3 slices deli roast beef and 1 or 2 slices whole-grain bread
- 6-ounce container of plain low-fat yogurt and 1 bowl oatmeal or high-fiber cereal

Rev Up Plan Recipes

Each recipe makes 2 8-ounce servings

Supreme Quick Blender Shake

1 cup 1% or fat-free milk
2 tablespoons low-fat vanilla yogurt
¾ cup instant apple-cinnamon oatmeal prepared with water in microwave
2 teaspoons peanut butter or other nut butter
2 teaspoons vanilla-flavored whey powder
A dash of cinnamon
6 ice cubes, crushed

Combine all ingredients in a blender and blend until smooth.

Strawberry Quick Blender Shake

½ cup low-fat vanilla yogurt
1 cup 1% or fat-free milk
2 teaspoons peanut butter or other nut butter
1 cup frozen unsweetened strawberries
2 teaspoons vanilla-flavored whey powder
6 ice cubes, crushed

Combine all ingredients in a blender and blend until smooth.

Fiber-Licious Quick Blender Shake

½ cup All-Bran® or Fiber One® cereal
1 cup 1% or fat-free milk
½ cup fresh or frozen unsweetened blueberries
1 tablespoon honey
2 teaspoons vanilla-flavored whey powder
6 ice cubes, crushed

Combine all ingredients in a blender and blend until smooth.

Mixed Berry Quick Blender Shake

¾ cup instant apple-cinnamon oatmeal prepared with water in microwave
¾ cup 1% or fat free milk
¾ cup mixed frozen unsweetened blueberries, strawberries, and raspberries
2 teaspoons vanilla-flavored whey powder
3 ice cubes, crushed

Combine all ingredients in a blender and blend until smooth.

Banana-Orange Quick Blender Shake

1 banana
½ cup low-fat vanilla yogurt
⅛ cup frozen orange juice concentrate
½ cup 1% or fat-free milk
2 teaspoons vanilla-flavored whey powder
6 ice cubes, crushed

Combine all ingredients in a blender and blend until smooth.

Nutter-Butter Quick Blender Shake

¾ cup low-fat vanilla yogurt
¾ cup 1% or fat-free milk
2 teaspoons peanut butter or other nut butter
1 medium banana
½ cup frozen unsweetened strawberries
2 teaspoons vanilla-flavored whey powder
4 ice cubes, crushed

Combine all ingredients in a blender and blend until smooth.

Berry-Melon Quick Blender Shake

⅔ cup frozen unsweetened strawberries
1 banana
½ cup cubed cantaloupe or other melon
¼ cup low-fat vanilla yogurt
¾ cup 1% milk
2 teaspoons vanilla-flavored whey powder
3 ice cubes, crushed

Combine all ingredients in a blender and blend until smooth.

Mainstream Plan

Follow this eating plan for the third and fourth weeks of your transformation. A seven day meal plan is presented and you can modify it with some of the listed alternative meals and also substitute similar food items for those listed. For the fifth and sixth weeks of your transformation, modify the menus to create an adaptation with a calorie balance for weight maintenance. A good calorie intake balance for weight control is 30 percent protein, 30 percent fat, and 40 percent carbohydrate calories. Of the carbohydrates, strive for about 80 percent from vegetables and 20 percent from fruit. You'll want to build your meals from various healthy foods that are low-glycemic (refer to the **Glycemic Index of Common Foods** table from Chapter 1). The **Food Portion and Serving Sizes** section in this chapter will help you learn to use the Nutrition Label on food products to aid you in determining calorie amounts of protein, fat, and carbohydrates. There are also tips on how to easily determine portion and serving sizes. By eating well consistently, you learn which foods best nourish and sustain you during stressful changes in your life. The **Eating Out** section in this chapter will help you plan and choose foods wisely when you are eating out, enabling to maintain your weight and health.

A good understanding of high- and low-carbohydrate foods and their effect on your body will help you make better food choices for health and well-being. Build your weight maintenance menus with a wide variety of fiber-rich foods (such as vegetables, fruits, whole grains), along with small amounts of healthy fats (such as nuts and olive oil), which is the best way to control your weight and blood sugar, vitamins and minerals. In effect, you are reducing saturated fat (the major source is fast foods), reducing refined sugar (soft drinks are a major source), and increasing fiber in your diet by reducing refined foods.

Last, but not least, you'll be adding more fitness activities to firm up your body, as well as exercises that specifically target your abdominal muscles.

Here are important points of the plan:

- Drink at least eight 8-ounce glasses of water throughout the day, plain or sparkling with a lemon or lime slice
- Eat every 3 hours to maintain your energy level
- Unless specified, eat moderately-sized food portions, don't fill a 12-inch plate to the edges with food
- Recipes follow the daily menus for the items marked with an asterisk (*)

- No need to count calories during the third and fourth weeks, however use your total daily calorie calculation and protein, fats, and carbohydrates percentages from your **My Ideal Daily Calorie Total** worksheet in Chapter 1 when planning your meals for the fifth and sixth weeks

- Continue cutting down or avoiding alcoholic drinks altogether, controlling excess and empty calories, while you reconstruct your eating plan

- Continue practicing and fine-tuning your selected stress reduction techniques

- Start adding in strengthening and aerobic conditioning fitness activities. Select from the fitness activities described in Chapter 3.

Weeks 3 and 4 Fitness Activities

o   Add in aerobic interval training fitness activities 2 to 3 days a week

o   Add in strengthening fitness activities 1 to 2 days a week

o   Add in abdominal core specific activities 1 day a week

Weeks 5 and 6 Fitness Activities

o   Perform aerobic or interval training fitness activities 3 days a week

o   Perform strengthening fitness activities 2 to 3 days a week

o   Perform abdominal core specific activities 2 to 3 days a week as part of your strengthening fitness activities

- Chart your progress every week on the fitness charts found in Chapter 4

Day 1

Breakfast
½ cup of ricotta cheese mixed with 1 tablespoon of chopped walnuts and 2 tablespoons of blueberries
1 cup water
Coffee or tea (black, green, or herbal)

Lunch
Deli roast beef sandwich on whole-grain bread or roll sandwich with 1 slice low-fat Swiss cheese, leaf lettuce, tomato slice, and 1 tablespoon sandwich spread or low-fat mayonnaise

Small bag of plain baked potato chips
Sparkling water with a slice of lemon or lime

Dinner
Herb Crusted Baked Cod*
1 cup Tabbouleh*
1 whole-grain sourdough roll
1 teaspoon Butter-and-Olive Oil Spread*
1 cup fresh berries sprinkled with cinnamon
Herbal iced tea or water

Snacks
Quick Blender Shake (recipe in **Rev Up Plan Recipes** section)
Small handful (1 ounce) pistachios

Day 2

Breakfast
½ cup fresh mixed chopped fruit (melons, banana, apple, berries), topped with
½ cup light vanilla-flavored yogurt and 2 tablespoons slivered almonds
½ whole wheat English muffin
1 cup skim milk
Tea (black, green, or herbal) or water

Lunch
Chicken wrap, with 1 medium flour tortilla filled with mixture of ⅓ cup cooked
chopped chicken, ½ cup shredded leaf lettuce, 2 medium tomato slices, 2 tablespoons fat-free mayonnaise and a dash of hot sauce
1 cup raw baby carrots
1 nectarine
Water or green tea

Dinner
Baked Spaghetti*
2 cups mixed salad greens
1 tablespoon low-fat Caesar dressing
1 whole-wheat roll
1 teaspoon Butter-and-Olive Oil Spread
Sparkling water
Frozen fruit bar or ½ cup fruit sorbet

Snacks
Trail mix made with 2 tablespoons raisins, 1 ounce unsalted mini twist pretzels (about 22), and 2 tablespoons sunflower seeds
1 medium apple or pear with 1 tablespoon peanut butter

Day 3

Breakfast
2" square Granola Bar*
1 banana
1 cup skim milk
Tea (black, green, or herbal) or water

Lunch
Grilled chicken Caesar salad
16 whole-wheat reduced-fat crackers
1 cup skim milk or water

Dinner
Lemony Shrimp or Salmon Fettuccine*
1 cup steamed green beans
Tossed green salad with shredded cheese
½ cup fruit sorbet
Green tea or water

Snack
¼ cup commercially- or home-prepared hummus
1 cup cut-up raw vegetables (broccoli, carrots, celery)
Whole-wheat pita bread wedges or crisp pita bread wedges toasted in the oven

Day 4

Breakfast
1 whole-wheat bagel, split in half and toasted, if desired
2 tablespoons peanut butter
1 medium orange or ½ grapefruit
1 cup skim milk
Coffee or tea (black, green, or herbal)

Lunch
1 cup vegetable soup
1 slice whole-grain bread or roll
1 ounce low-fat cheese
3 raw carrot sticks (3")
3 raw celery sticks (4")
Water

Dinner
Broiled or grilled chicken breasts
1 cup of basmati rice (brown or white)
1 cup cooked Herbed Vegetables*
Small Mediterranean Chopped Salad*
Green or black tea or water

Snacks
6-ounce container of flavored or plain low-fat yogurt
Small handful (1 ounce) almonds
1 medium whole fruit

Day 5

Breakfast
1 scrambled egg, sprinkled with 1 ounce of low-fat shredded cheddar cheese
½ whole-wheat English muffin
6 ounces orange juice or grapefruit juice
1 cup skim milk
Tea (black, green, or herbal) or water

Lunch
1 whole-wheat pita stuffed with 1 cup shredded lettuce, 2 tomato slices, 1 ounce feta or cheddar cheese, 1 teaspoon of sliced black or green olives, and 2 tablespoons fat-free ranch dressing
1 nectarine or peach
Sparkling water with a slice of lemon or lime

Dinner
Stir-Fry Beef or Chicken with Broccoli and Carrots*
1 cup brown rice
2 cups mixed salad greens

1 tablespoon fat-free ranch dressing
2 cantaloupe wedges
Water

Snacks
Three cups of popcorn, air-popped or light microwave variety (no trans-fat, if possible)
¾ cup low-fat plain yogurt with 2 tablespoons granola cereal

Day 6

Breakfast
1 breakfast burrito (1 scrambled egg, picante salsa, and low-fat shredded cheese in a whole-wheat flour tortilla)
1 slice whole-grain toast
1 teaspoon Butter-and-Olive Oil Spread
6 ounces apple or grape juice
Tea (black, green, or herbal) or water

Lunch
1 Mediterranean Pizza Wedge*
Small tossed salad with extra-virgin olive oil and lemon juice dressing
1 banana
Water

Dinner
Better Burger*
½ cup green beans
Small Greek Salad*
Green or black tea or water

Snacks
A medium bunch of grapes
Small handful (1 ounce) of peanuts

Day 7

Breakfast
Cold whole-grain cereal with ½ to ¾ cup of low-fat milk and ½ cup slice strawberries

1 slice whole-grain bread
1 teaspoon Butter-and-Olive Oil Spread
Tea (black, green, or herbal) or water

Lunch
Deli turkey sandwich on whole-grain bread or roll sandwich with 1 slice low-fat Swiss cheese, leaf lettuce, tomato slice, and 1 tablespoon sandwich spread or low-fat mayonnaise
Small tossed salad with extra-virgin olive oil and vinegar dressing
1 banana
Water

Dinner
Sirloin beef tips and noodles (4 ounces beef and ½ cup noodles) from prepared package
1 whole-grain dinner roll or bread
1 teaspoon Butter-and-Olive Oil Spread
1 cup steamed green beans
1 cup sliced strawberries
Green or black tea or water

Snacks
Hard-boiled egg
Small bag of plain baked potato chips

Alternative meals and snacks

Brunch
1 slice of Spanish Frittata*
1 tablespoon salsa
1 slice whole-grain bread
1 teaspoon Butter-and-Olive Oil Spread
Mixed sliced berries, fresh or frozen (strawberries, blueberries, blackberries, raspberries)
Water or green or black tea

Lunch
1 cup of Chicken Noodle and Brown Rice Soup*
5 saltine crackers

Three-Bean Salad*
1 cup skim milk

Dinner
1 cup Andalusian Lentil Stew*
2 slices of crusty Italian or French bread
Extra-virgin olive oil for dipping bread, if desired
Small Mediterranean chopped salad*
Water or green or black tea

Sandwich variation
1 Mediterranean Steak Sandwich*

Snacks

- Small bunch of grapes, 3 graham crackers, and 1 cup of low-fat milk
- 1 slice date-nut bread topped with 1 teaspoon low-fat cream cheese and ½ ounce raisins; and 1 cup low-fat milk
- 1 ounce baked tortilla chips dipped in 2 tablespoons low-fat refried beans and 2 tablespoons salsa
- ½ cantaloupe filled with ¾ cup low-fat lemon yogurt
- 1 cup warmed low-fat milk flavored with a dash of almond extract, 1 banana, and 1 ounce peanuts
- ½ cup soy nuts and ½ cup canned mixed fruit, low syrup
- 1 cup low-sodium canned bean soup, 1 slice whole-wheat bread, and ½ cup canned tangerine segments, drained or 1 whole tangerine, peeled into segments
- ¼ cup chickpeas, rinsed, drained, and seasoned with garlic powder, paprika, and lemon juice; and 1 cup grapefruit juice
- 1 large romaine lettuce leaf wrapped around 2 ounces leftover chicken, fish, or beans, ½ ounce low-fat cheddar cheese, and 1 teaspoon low-fat ranch dressing

Pre-Workout
Quality carbohydrates are needed for energy. Drinking plenty of fluids keeps you hydrated.

- ½ cup all-fruit sorbet, ¼ cup berries, and 1 cup water

- ¼ cup snack mix made with unsalted whole-wheat pretzels, dried fruit and toasted almonds; 1 orange; and 1 cup water
- 1 small to medium whole-wheat bagel topped with 1 teaspoon fat-free cream cheese, 1 lettuce leaf, and 2 pineapple rings; and 1 cup water

Post-Workout
Replenish carbohydrates and fluids. Add protein to build muscle.

- 2 fig bars, 1 cup low-fat milk, and 1 medium piece of whole fruit
- 1 ounce of low-fat cheese, cut into strips and placed on 6 low-fat whole-wheat crackers, 1 medium apple, and 1 cup of water
- 3 ounces chunk light tuna on 6 low-fat whole-wheat crackers, spread with 1 teaspoon low-calorie or low-fat mayonnaise and 1 teaspoon pickle relish; and 6 ounce orange juice or grapefruit juice
- ¾ cup low-fat vanilla yogurt with 2 teaspoons almonds and 2 teaspoons raisins; 1 small banana; 2 graham crackers; and 1 cup water

Mainstream Recipes

Herb Crusted Baked Cod

8 ounces Cod fish, fresh or frozen, thawed
3 tablespoons honey
½ cup herb-flavored bread stuffing
Nonstick cooking spray
1-quart size plastic storage bag

Preheat oven to 375° F.

1. Wash cod.
2. Spray baking dish with nonstick spray.
3. Brush honey on the cod.
4. Discard any extra honey.
5. Place bread stuffing in the plastic bag and crush it to crumb texture.
6. Place cod in bag with stuffing and coat cod.
7. Place in pan and bake until done, approximately 10 minutes.
8. The cod could also be grilled. Prepare grill, wrap the cod in foil and grill.

Serves 2

Tabbouleh

¾ cup bulgur
Cold water
½ medium cucumber, seeded and coarsely chopped
½ cup snipped fresh parsley
6 green onions, sliced
2 medium tomatoes, chopped
¼ cup extra-virgin olive oil
¼ cup lemon juice
1 clove garlic, minced
⅛ teaspoon pepper

1. In a medium-sized bowl, place the bulgur and cover it with cold water and soak for 20 minutes. Rinse bulgur in a colander. Drain well.

2. In a separate bowl, combine bulgur, cucumber, parsley, onions, and tomatoes.

3. In a screw top jar, combine oil, lemon juice, mint, garlic, salt, and pepper. Cover; shake to mix. Pour over bulgur mixture. Toss to coat.

4. Cover and chill 4 to 24 hours.

Serves 6

Butter-and-Olive Oil Spread

½ stick of softened butter
¼ cup of extra virgin olive oil

1. Blend together the butter and oil.

2. Store in an opaque, sealed container in the refrigerator.

Makes ½ cup

Baked Spaghetti

½ pound lean ground beef or turkey
1 small onion, diced
1 box (7-ounce) whole-wheat elbow macaroni
1 jar (15-ounce) spaghetti sauce
4 tablespoons Parmesan cheese

Preheat oven to 350° F.

1. In a nonstick frying pan, cook ground beef or turkey until browned (beef) or dark white (turkey). Add onion and cook until soft and translucent. Drain well.

2. Fill a large pot three-fourths full with water and bring to a boil. Add the pasta and cook al dente (tender), 10 to 12 minutes, or according to the package directions. Drain the pasta thoroughly.

3.   Add the cooked pasta to the meat and onions. Add the spaghetti sauce and stir so that the ingredients are evenly mixed. Spoon the mixture into a baking dish. Bake for 25 to 35 minutes or until bubbly.

4.   Divide the spaghetti among 4 plates. Sprinkle each serving with 1 tablespoon Parmesan cheese.

Serves 4

Granola Bars

1 cup granola or crunchy Kashi™ Crunch cereal
1 cup quick-cooking rolled oats
1 cup chopped walnuts
½ cup unbleached all-purpose or whole-wheat flour
½ cup raisins
1 beaten egg
⅓ cup honey
⅓ cup extra-virgin olive oil
¼ cup packed brown sugar
½ teaspoon ground cinnamon

Preheat oven to 325° F.

1.   Line an 8 x 8 x 2-inch baking dish with foil. Grease the foil; set pan aside.

2.   In a mixing bowl combine granola, oats, nuts, flour, and raisins. Stir in egg, honey, oil, brown sugar, and cinnamon. Press evenly into the prepared pan.

3.   Bake in a 325° F oven for 30 to 35 minutes or until lightly browned around the edges.

4.   Cool. Use foil to remove from pan. Cut into 2" bars.

Makes sixteen 2" square bars

Lemony Shrimp or Salmon Fettuccine

1 pound whole-wheat fettuccine pasta
1 teaspoon extra-virgin olive oil
1 10-ounce package of frozen green peas

1 jar (16-ounce) low-fat or reduced-calorie Alfredo sauce
8-ounces deveined, peeled shrimp or 8-ounce fresh or frozen salmon fillet, sliced into thin 2 x 1-inch pieces
⅓ cup finely chopped fresh dill
1 tablespoon freshly grated lemon zest

1. Bring a large pot of water and 1 teaspoon olive oil to a boil. Add pasta and cook, stirring often, 7 minutes. Add peas; boil 5 to 6 minutes until pasta is firm tender.

2. Meanwhile, stir Alfredo sauce in a medium saucepan over medium-low heat 3 minutes, or until simmering. Add shrimp or salmon, and stirring gently, simmer 3 to 5 minutes until shrimp or fish is tender. Cover; remove from heat.

3. Remove ½ cup cooking water from pasta pot. Drain pasta and peas; return to pot. Add sauce, reserved cooking water, dill and lemon zest. Gently turn with spoon to mix and coat.

4. Pour into a serving dish and serve.

Serves 6

Herbed Vegetables

1 9- or 10-ounce package (2 cups) frozen vegetables of your choice
Water
¼ cup chopped onion
¼ teaspoon dried thyme, oregano, basil, rosemary, or dill, crushed
1 tablespoon extra-virgin olive oil
¼ teaspoon salt

1. In a medium saucepan, cook the vegetables according to package directions. Drain and put in a serving dish.

2. In a small saucepan, cook the onion and herbs in oil until the onion is tender.

3. Add the onion mixture and salt to the vegetables; toss gently to coat the vegetables. Serve warm.

Serves 4

Mediterranean Chopped Salad

1 medium romaine lettuce, shredded
1 cucumber, peeled and diced into ¼-inch cubes
1 red bell pepper, diced into ¼-inch cubes
2 tablespoons chopped red onion
2 tablespoons finely chopped fresh parsley
1 tomato, diced into ¼-inch cubes
1 tablespoon lemon juice
2 tablespoons extra-virgin olive oil

1. Mix all ingredients together in a large nonmetallic bowl and serve.

Serves 4

Stir-Fry Beef or Chicken with Broccoli and Carrots

1 pound boneless beef sirloin steak or top round steak, sliced into thin strips
or 1 pound chicken strips
¼ cup cider vinegar
3 tablespoons reduced-sodium soy sauce
1 tablespoon cornstarch
½ teaspoon ground ginger
⅓ cup water
1 tablespoon sesame oil or extra-virgin olive oil
2 cloves garlic, minced
3 medium carrots cut into 1" julienne strips
1 cup broccoli florets
1 medium onion, cut into thin wedges

1. Combine vinegar, soy sauce, cornstarch, ginger, and ⅓ cup water in a small bowl. Set aside.

2. Preheat a large skillet over high heat and add oil (add more oil as necessary during cooking). Add carrots and stir-fry 2 minutes. Add broccoli and onion; continue to stir fry about 3 minutes more or until crisp-tender. Remove vegetables from the skillet.

3. Add half of the beef or chicken to the hot skillet. Stir-fry for 2 to 3 minutes or until done. Remove. Repeat with remaining beef or chicken. Return all beef or chicken to skillet. Push from center of skillet.

4. Stir sauce and add to center of skillet. Cook and stir until bubbly. Cook and stir 2 minutes more.

5. Stir in vegetables. Cover and cook for 1 minute or until hot.

6. Serve over hot cooked rice.

Serves 4

Mediterranean Pizza Wedges

1 6-inch whole-wheat pita bread
1 tablespoon extra-virgin olive oil
1 small Roma tomato, thinly sliced
⅓ cup thinly sliced spinach or artichoke hearts
2 tablespoons crumbled feta cheese or shredded mozzarella cheese

Preheat oven to 425° F.

1. Drizzle oil on top of bread.

2. Layer tomato slices, spinach or artichoke hearts on top.

3. Sprinkle top with cheese.

4. Bake pizza at 425° F for 8 to 10 minutes or until crisp and warmed through.

5. Cut into 6 wedges and serve.

Serves 1 (6 wedges)

Greek Salad

3 cups torn romaine lettuce
1½ cups torn spinach
1 medium tomato, chopped
½ of a small cucumber, thinly sliced
½ cup crumbled feta cheese
2 green onions, sliced
2 tablespoons sliced pitted Kalamata or black olives
½ cup Garlic Vinaigrette*

1. In a large salad bowl, toss together lettuce and spinach.

2. Arrange meat, tomato, cucumber, feta cheese, green onions, radishes, and olives over greens.

3. Drizzle with garlic vinaigrette.

Serves 3

Garlic Vinaigrette

½ cup extra-virgin olive oil
⅓ cup balsamic vinegar
1 tablespoon sugar
2 large cloves garlic, minced
1 teaspoon Dijon-style mustard
⅛ teaspoon pepper

1. In a screw-top jar, mix oil, vinegar, sugar, garlic, mustard, and pepper.

2. Cover and shake well. Store in the refrigerator up to 2 weeks. Shake before serving.

Makes ¾ cup (twelve 1-tablespoon servings)

Oriental Chicken

2 boneless, skinless chicken breasts
1 tablespoon cornstarch
1 tablespoon brown sugar
¼ teaspoon dried oregano, crushed
1 clove crushed garlic
½ teaspoon sesame oil
1½ teaspoons reduced-sodium soy sauce
¾ cup white wine or water
1 teaspoon sunflower seeds
2 pineapple rings

1. Pierce chicken breasts with a fork.

2. Mix cornstarch, brown sugar, oregano, garlic, sesame oil, soy sauce, and white wine together.

3. Pour the liquid mixture over the chicken.

4. Cover and microwave on high for about 10 minutes or until done.

5. While chicken is cooking, spray a pan with cooking spray and sauté the pineapple over medium heat.

6. Before serving, top each breast with pineapple ring and ½ teaspoon of sunflower seeds.

Serves 2

Better Burger

¾ **pound ground turkey breast or extra-lean ground beef**
¼ **cup chopped onion**
2 **teaspoons Worcestershire sauce**
2 **whole-grain buns**

1. Combine the ground turkey breast or beef, chopped onion and Worcestershire sauce in a large bowl.

2. Mix well.

3. Divide turkey mixture into equal portions.

4. Prepare grill, or preheat broiler.

5. Grill burgers until golden brown and cooked through and white (turkey) or gray (beef) inside—about 7 to 10 minutes per side.

6. In the meantime, toast buns.

7. Put burger on bun and add toppings of choice.

Serves 2

Mediterranean Steak Sandwiches

Seasoning:
1 **tablespoon lemon juice**
1½ **teaspoons dried basil**
1½ **teaspoons garlic powder**
1½ **teaspoons dried oregano**
½ **teaspoon salt**
⅛ **teaspoon pepper**

2 **beef rib eye steaks, cut 1-inch thick (about 1½ pounds)**
1 **tablespoon extra-virgin olive oil**

4 6-inch pita breads, warmed
2 tablespoons crumbled feta cheese
1 tablespoon chopped pitted Kalamata or black olives

1. Combine seasoning ingredients; press onto beef steaks.

2. Heat oil in large nonstick skillet over medium heat until hot. Place steaks in skillet; cook 12 to 15 minutes for medium rare to medium doneness, turning occasionally. Sprinkle with lemon juice.

3. Slice steaks; place on top of pitas. Sprinkle with cheese and olives.

Serves 4

Three-Bean Salad

1 15-ounce can chickpeas (garbanzo beans)
1 15-ounce can kidney beans
1 15-ounce can black beans
2 cloves garlic, minced
2 tablespoons finely chopped fresh parsley or ½ tablespoon dried parsley, crushed
2 tablespoons lemon juice
2 tablespoons extra-virgin olive oil

1. Drain beans thoroughly. Mix beans together in a salad bowl.

2. In a small bowl, combine garlic, parsley, lemon juice, and olive oil.

3. Pour the dressing over the beans, toss gently and serve.

Serves 8

Andalusian Lentil Stew

1 cup dry lentils
1 cup chopped onions
2 clove garlic, minced
1 tablespoon extra-virgin olive oil
4 cups beef stock
1 7.5-ounce can diced tomatoes
1 tablespoon Worcestershire sauce
¼ teaspoon dried thyme or oregano, crushed

¼ teaspoon pepper
⅛ teaspoon ground cumin
1 bay leaf
½ cup chopped carrot
½ cup chopped celery
½ **pound fully cooked turkey kielbasa sausage links, cut in 1-inch thick slices**

1. Rinse lentils and set aside.

2. In a large soup pot, cook onion and garlic in hot oil until tender, but not brown.

3. Stir in the lentils, beef stock, undrained tomatoes, Worcestershire sauce, thyme or oregano, pepper, cumin, and bay leaf. Bring to boiling; reduce heat. Cover and simmer for 15 minutes.

4. Add carrot and celery. Return to boiling; reduce heat. Simmer for 15 to 20 minutes more or till the lentils and vegetables are tender.

5. Stir in sausage slices; heat through. Remove and discard bay leaf.

6. Serve with crusty bread dipped in extra-virgin olive oil.

Serves 4

Spanish Frittata

3 tablespoons olive oil
1 large russet potato (about 12 ounces), peeled, thinly sliced
1 medium onion, thinly sliced
1 large red bell pepper, seeded and thinly sliced
1 tablespoon chopped fresh thyme or 1 teaspoon dried
6 large eggs
½ cup grated Parmesan cheese
Salt and pepper to taste

1. Heat 2 tablespoons oil in 12-inch nonstick skillet over medium heat. Layer half of potato, onion, and bell pepper slices in skillet. Season with salt and pepper.

2. Repeat layering and seasoning. Cover and cook until potatoes and vegetables are tender, stirring and turning frequently with a spatula, about 20 minutes. Sprinkle with thyme. Cool slightly.

3. Whisk eggs in a large bowl to blend. Season with salt and pepper. Add potato mixture to eggs.

4. Wipe skillet clean. Heat 1 tablespoon oil in same skillet over medium-low heat. Pour egg mixture into skillet; sprinkle with cheese. Cover and cook until eggs are just set, about 10 minutes.

5. Slide frittata onto a platter.

Serves 3

Chicken Noodle and Brown Rice Soup

1 2½-pound chicken cut up, use neck and livers
3 stalks celery with leaves, cut up
2 medium carrots, cut up
1 large onion, cut up
2 tablespoons snipped fresh cilantro
1 teaspoon salt
½ teaspoon dried thyme, sage, or basil, crushed
¼ teaspoon pepper
2 bay leaves
8 to 10 cups cold water
1 cup whole-wheat egg noodles
1 tablespoon snipped fresh cilantro
1 cup cooked brown rice

1. In a large stock pot, place chicken pieces, celery, carrots, onion, cilantro, salt, herbs, pepper, and bay leaves. Add water.

2. Bring to boiling; reduce heat. Cover and simmer for 2 hours.

3. Remove chicken and let cool. When meat is cool enough to handle, remove meat from bones and put meat back into soup pot. Discard bones.

4. Bring soup back to a boil. Stir in the egg noodles and cilantro. Return to boil; reduce heat.

5. Cover and simmer about 8 minutes or till noodles are done. Stir in the cooked rice.

Serves 8 to 12

Custom Meal Planner

Create your own custom meals for the fifth and sixth weeks using the following meal planning worksheet. You may wish to photocopy and enlarge the worksheet to make it easier to write in your meal entries and read them. Make as many copies as you need. Consider your total daily calorie calculation and protein, fat, and carbohydrate percentages when planning your meals. Chapter 4 has a more detailed Nutrition Log where you can chart the calorie composition and macronutrient percentages of your meals.

Custom Meal Planner

	Breakfast	Lunch	Dinner	Snack
Sunday				
Monday				
Tuesday				
Wednesday				
Thursday				
Friday				
Saturday				

Food Portion and Serving Sizes

The Nutrition Facts label on food products makes it easy for you to know what is in the food you eat. Sections on the label consist of Serving Size Information, Amount of Calories per Serving and Calories from Fat, a Nutrition Panel, and a Nutrition Reference footnote panel. The Nutrition Panel lists nutrients that are most important to the health of people today, such as Total Fat (grams), Saturated Fat (grams), Trans Fat (grams), Polyunsaturated Fat (grams), Monounsaturated Fat (grams), Cholesterol (milligrams), Sodium (milligrams), Potassium (milligrams), Total Carbohydrate (grams), Dietary Fiber (grams), Sugars (grams), and Protein (grams). The Percentage Daily Value shows you the percentage (or how much) of the recommended dietary amount of a nutrient is in one serving of the food based on the nutrition values in the Nutrition Reference footnote. The Percentage Daily Values (% Daily Value) of each amount are based on a 2,000-calorie diet. The Percentage Daily Values of the vitamins and minerals are based on the Food and Nutrition Board's Recommended Dietary Allowances (RDA). For example, if a product has listed the % Daily Value for vitamin C as 2 percent and the RDA is 75 mg, then this product is providing 12 mg of vitamin C (0.02 multiplied by 75 mg equals 1.5 mg). Another example, if calcium is listed as 30 percent and the RDA is 1,000 mg, and then this product provides 300 mg.

The Nutrition Reference footnote has nutritional data for Total Fat including types of fat such as Saturated or Trans; Cholesterol; Sodium; Total Carbohydrate; and Dietary Fiber based on a diet that is approximately 60 percent carbohydrates, 30 percent fats, and 10 percent protein. It lists the data for a 2,000-calorie-a-day diet and a 2,500-calorie-a-day diet. Data on this footnote do not change from food product to food product; it shows dietary advice.

Here's how to use the information on these labels to make wise decisions on portion size. Say, for example, that an 11.5-ounce can of vegetable juice states that the serving size is 1 can, the number of calories for this serving is 70, and the total carbohydrate amount is 15 grams. If you were reducing your carbohydrate intake, you could drink half of the serving amount, taking in 35 calories with 7.5 grams of carbohydrates. Now, what about a 20-ounce bottle of a soft drink? The number of calories per serving shows about 140 calories. However, the serving size is 2.5 servings. If you drink the entire bottle, you've taken in 350 calories! This may not be the caloric amount you had in mind if you thought the whole bottle was one serving! Look at the Nutrition Facts label to learn the *size* of the serving and the *number* of servings.

Standard Serving Sizes

The U.S. Department of Agriculture's (USDA) *Dietary Guidelines for Americans* sets forth serving size standards based on typical portion sizes and the nutritional content of foods. It describes serving *units* for each food group, such as ½ cup cooked vegetables and 1 cup raw leafy vegetables, to make it easy for consumers to make healthful food choices. These servings units cover simple food items, such as fruits, vegetables, and plain grain products.

Generally, standard serving sizes are as follows:

Grain Products (bread, cereal, rice, and pasta)

- 1 slice of bread
- 1 ounce of ready-to-eat cereal
- ½ cup of cooked cereal, rice, or pasta

Vegetables and Fruits

- 1 cup of raw leafy vegetables
- ½ cup of other vegetables—cooked or chopped raw
- ¾ cup of vegetable juice
- 1 medium apple, banana, orange
- ½ cup of chopped, cooked, or canned fruit
- ¾ cup of fruit juice

Protein (meat, poultry, fish, dry beans, eggs, and nuts) and Dairy (milk, yogurt, and cheese)

- 2 to 3 ounces of cooked lean meat, poultry, or fish
- ½ cup of cooked dry beans or 1 egg counts as 1 ounce of lean meat; 2 tablespoons of peanut butter or ⅓ cup of nuts count as 1 ounce of meat
- 1 cup of milk or yogurt
- 1½ ounces of natural cheese
- 2 ounces of processed cheese

Determining Food Serving Sizes

It is so easy to overestimate how much food makes up a serving size. The most important thing is to be able to eyeball portion sizes and know how much you are really eating. There are three methods that may work for you: the comparison method, the pre-measured method, and the hand method.

1. **Comparison Method:** Compare how much of what you are eating with a familiar object. Here are a few comparisons:

1 ounce cheese	A pair of dice
3 ounces of meat	A deck of cards
½ cup mashed potatoes	An ice cream scoop
1 medium potato	A computer mouse
½ cup serving of grapes	A light bulb
1 serving of fruit	A tennis ball
1 serving of pasta	A hockey puck
1 serving of bread	A cassette tape
1 tablespoon of peanut butter	A walnut
¼ cup serving	A golf ball
2½ ounce bagel	Length of a credit card
6 ounces of juice	Small yogurt container

2. **Pre-Measured Method:** Using a set of measuring spoons, a glass measuring cup for liquids, a set of measuring cups for dry foods, and a kitchen scale for weighing raw fruits and vegetables, meat, and cheese, you pre-measure all your food portions. You will be surprised to see the actual amount of a serving size of food on your dinner plate or in your cereal bowl.

   Weigh meat, poultry, and fish after cooking. In restaurants, the menu lists the precooked weight of the meat, so use this conversion rule to convert raw weight into cooked weight:

   - Meat with bone: 5 raw ounces equals 3 ounces cooked (a standard serving size is 3 ounces).

   - Meat without bone: 4 raw ounces equals 3 ounces cooked.

   Examples of pre-measured quantities:

   Bagel

       Small   2 ounces

Medium	3 ounces
Large	4 ounces

Bread Roll

Small	1.5 ounces
Medium	1.8 ounces
Large	2.7 ounces
Extra large	4.5 ounces

Grapes

Small bunch	4 ounces
Large bunch	8 ounces
Extra-large bunch	16 ounces

Bananas

Small	5 ounces
Medium	6 ounces
Large	8 ounces

3. **Hand Method:** Use your hand to gauge portion size. Here are some approximate measurements based on an average-size woman's hand:

Thumb volume	1 ounce or 1 tablespoon
	Good estimate for nut butter, spreads and dips, mayonnaise, oils, salad dressings, sour cream, cream cheese
Thumb tip	1 teaspoon
Finger length	Diameter of 1 serving of fruit
Fist volume (clenched fist)	1 cup or 2 servings of pasta, cereal, cooked vegetables, or 1 serving of raw vegetables
Palm area	3-ounce serving of meat, fish, poultry
Handful	1 serving of nuts
Two handfuls	1 serving of most snack foods

Eating Out

You can make healthful food choices when dining out. Many fast-food chains and restaurants provide nutritional information for their customers at the establishment or on their Web sites. This information can help you make a healthful food choice when your only eating choice is at a restaurant. Some pocket calorie, fat, and carbohydrate counter guides have a section on the most popular fast-food chains and restaurants. Keeping one with you will increase your ability to choose more healthful foods when dining out.

Many, if not most, restaurants serve oversize portions, which equate to extra food and an increased amount of calories, fat, cholesterol, and sodium. A 10-inch plate of spaghetti is not a single serving size of ½ cup. To keep your portion sizes at a reasonable level:

- Order menu items a la carte. This gives you a variety of foods in smaller quantities.

- Ask if you can have a lunch portion, even if you're eating dinner. Or simply request a smaller portion.

- Split a meal with a companion, particularly when you know the restaurant serves larger portions.

- Request a to-go container when the meal arrives. Immediately place half of the food into the container for another day's meal.

- Eat only until your hunger is satisfied. If you're tempted to clean your plate, ask your server to remove the dishes.

At Restaurants

Read through the menu and select the items that are lower in saturated fat and calories. Read the description of the menu item. If none is available, ask your server what's in the meal and how it's prepared. Choose dishes based on fruits, vegetables, and whole grains rather than those based on meat. Plant-based foods are naturally low in fat and calories and are good sources of vitamins, minerals, and fiber. Fish and seafood also are good meal options.

You can find healthful options within each course of the meal. Here's how to do it:

- **Appetizers:** Choose appetizers with vegetables, fruits, or fish. Tomato juice, fresh fruit compote, and shrimp cocktail served with lemon are healthful options. Avoid fried or breaded appetizers.

- **Soup:** Choose broth-based or tomato-based soups, such as minestrone, vegetable, or gazpacho. Creamed soups, chowders, puréed soups and sometimes fruit soups can contain heavy cream or egg yolks. Ask your server for the soup's ingredients to find out for sure.

- **Salad:** Order lettuce or spinach salad with dressing on the side, preferably oil and vinegar or vinaigrette. Caesar, Greek, and taco salads tend to be higher in fat and calories. Similarly, chef salads can be high in fat, cholesterol, and calories because of the added dressing, cheese, eggs, and meat.

- **Bread:** Choose whole-grain breads, rolls, breadsticks, crackers, or bagels. Muffins, garlic toast, and croissants have more calories and fat. If you have a basket of bread at your table, take one piece and ask your server to remove the basket. Use only small amounts of added fat—such as margarine, butter, or olive oil—or none at all.

- **Side dish:** Choose steamed or sautéed vegetables rather than a baked potato, boiled new potatoes, or rice. Skip the French fries, potato chips, onion rings, or mayonnaise-based salads. Ask that the vegetables be served without butter or cream sauces.

- **Entrée:** Look for descriptions that indicate lower-fat preparations, such as London broil, grilled chicken breast, lemon-baked fish, or broiled shish kebabs. Avoid items with high-fat descriptors, such as prime rib of beef, veal parmigiana, stuffed shrimp, fried chicken, fettuccine Alfredo, filet mignon with béarnaise sauce, shrimp tempura, or fried rice. Choose pasta primavera or linguine with red tomato or clam sauce. Skip pasta with meat or cheese stuffing or sauces that contain bacon, butter, cream, or eggs.

- **Dessert:** Finish the main meal before ordering dessert. By the time you're done, you may not even want dessert. If you do order dessert, split it with your companions or take half of it home. Tasty and healthful dessert options include fresh fruit, gelatin, angel food cake, sorbet, or sherbet.

- **Beverages:** Many soft drinks contain a large number of calories. Instead, order water, unsweetened iced tea, sparkling water, or mineral water with a twist of lemon. For a hot drink, try black, decaffeinated coffee or black or green tea, minus the sugar and other extras. Remember, too, that alcohol also contains many calories, and it may further stimulate your appetite and decrease your inhibitions about overeating. Enjoy these drinks in moderation.

Chinese, Italian, and Mexican Meal Choices

Watch out for high sodium and saturated fat in these meals. Make your selections from some of the popular dishes that have lower sodium and saturated fat.

Chinese choices:

- Steamed rice instead of fried-rice with your meals (½ cup rice is a serving size)
- Szechuan shrimp, without peanuts
- Stir-fried vegetables, shrimp with garlic sauce
- Vegetable lo mein
- Chicken chow mein
- Beef and broccoli

Italian choices (if you are choosing pasta, rather than broiled or grilled meat):
- A salad with half the dressing, if the dressing is served over the salad
- Minestrone and fagioli soups
- Spaghetti with marinara (tomato sauce) or meat sauce
- Linguini with red clam or white clam sauce

Mexican choices:

- Garden salad, with dressing on the side
- Jicama salad with vinaigrette
- Chicken, shrimp, or vegetable fajitas, without the beans, sour cream, and guacamole
- Grilled fish or chicken with tomatillo sauce

At Buffets

With buffets, large amounts of food and the freedom to go back for a second or third helping may lead to excess. To limit the amount of food you eat, survey the entire buffet line, and then decide what you want and take only that. Make salad minus the high-fat dressings and toppings, such as cheese and croutons, your first course. Then, go back for an entrée. Fill up on vegetables that don't have added butter or sauces.

At Fast-Food Restaurants

The nutritional value of fast foods, from cheeseburger to leanburgers to pizzas to tacos, can vary greatly. The majority of fast foods are high in calories, saturated fat, cholesterol, sodium, and sugar. Fried foods such as French fries and crispy chicken breasts are high in fat. However, fast-food restaurants are expanding their food choices to include healthy foods such as salads, salad bars, low-fat meat, whole-wheat breads, low-carbohydrate sandwiches, low-fat sandwiches, low-fat milk products, low-calorie foods, and vegetable oils. Avoid condiments such as special sauces, mayonnaise, cheese sauce, salad dressing, tartar sauce, and ketchup. They are high in fat and sugar. Some healthy food choices include:

- Grilled chicken
- Whole-wheat rolls
- Fruit or fruit and yogurt
- Salad with dressing on the side or fat-free salad dressing
- Single hamburger (regular or childrens's size)
- Low-fat deli sandwiches on wheat bread or on pita bread
- Wraps on whole-wheat tortillas without the dressing
- Water or low-fat milk

At a Pizza Chain

Some dietitians claim that pizza is a nutritious meal by itself, because it contains a grain, vegetable, dairy, and meat product. But it also comes with a high saturated fat count. The typical serving size of pizza varies from two slices to three slices, or approximately 9 ounces, depending on the restaurant and type of pizza. Make your selections from some of the popular pizza toppings that have lower sodium and saturated fat:

- Select vegetable toppings.
- If you must have meat, select chicken or ham. If not chicken or ham, make pepperoni your next choice; it is leaner than pork, sausage, and beef.
- Order your pizza with half the cheese or no cheese. Skip the extra cheese.

- Order a salad to go along with your pizza. Ask for the dressing on the side.

At the Airport

Airports can be stressful places. Eat because you're hungry, not because you're stressed, bored, or trying to kill time. If you're anxious or have time to spare, take a walk. Airports usually have plenty of room for a brisk walk. Here are some pointers:

- **Check out your dining options.** There are a lot more options, with more healthful choices. Skip the hot dog and pizza counters and look for eateries that serve fruit, soup, sushi, and sandwiches or wraps.

- **Order ahead.** If your flight includes a meal, request a special diet when you make your reservation. You might be able to choose a low-salt or low-fat option, or a diet or vegetarian plate. And when the beverage cart rolls your way, ask for water or juice instead of alcohol or soda.

- **Go Prepared.** Take along your own food if you're leaving or arriving very early or late when eateries are likely to be closed. You don't have to pack a picnic. A whole-wheat bagel or crackers, a piece of fruit, granola bar, juice box, or cut-up cheese and vegetables can save you from feeling starved.

At the Office

If you only have fifteen minutes for lunch between meetings, skip the vending machine. Keep your desk drawer stocked with nutritious foods that contribute to a healthy diet. When stocking your drawer, consider office foods that don't require refrigeration and can keep well for a month or so:

- Soup you can microwave
- Nuts and seeds
- Whole grain, low-fat crackers (Melba toast, Wasa®, low-fat Triscuit®)
- Whole-wheat pretzels
- Cheese and cracker snack packs
- Microwavable low-fat popcorn
- Granola bars

- Applesauce in cups
- Juice boxes (100% juice, vitamin C-rich, or vegetable juice)

Keep some take-out menus from nearby restaurants in your office for when you have to work late or have a little more time for lunch.

In the Car

Keep some of the same snacks you have in your office in your car. When you're dashing from one activity to another or stuck in traffic, they come in handy.

Chapter 3

Fitness

Fitness leads to an improved sense of well-being, improved appearance, weight control, and increased stamina and strength. It also reduces your risk of developing chronic diseases, such as high blood pressure, hardening of the arteries, and diabetes.

Most experts agree that overall fitness consists of three areas:

- **Flexibility:** The ability to move joints and use muscles through their full range of motion. Stretching is a flexibility exercise.

- **Aerobic fitness:** The conditioning of your heart and lungs. It increases the amount of oxygen that is delivered to your muscles, which allows them to work longer. Walking is a type of aerobic exercise.

- **Strengthening:** Muscle strengthening includes building more powerful muscles and increasing how long you can use them (endurance). Weight lifting builds stronger muscles and strengthens bones, while push-ups build endurance.

Before starting any fitness or exercise program, consult your doctor for a complete checkup. Exercising should not hurt. Exercising may cause minor soreness only. If more discomfort is felt during exercise, stop immediately and consult your doctor.

Flexibility Fitness

Stretching elongates your muscles, which keeps them flexible. Stretching helps you avoid muscle aches and pains that may result from your aerobic and strength fitness programs. It also increases your balance and stability, enhances blood circulation, and helps relaxation. Stretching before and after aerobic exercise (even walking) and muscle strengthening help you feel better, avoid injury, and prevent aches and pains.

For extensive flexibility fitness, you may want to participate in activities that include stretching, such as dance, martial arts (aikido or karate), tai chi, or yoga.

Aerobic Fitness

Aerobic fitness burns fat and calories, and allows muscles to work at a steady rate with a constant supply of oxygen-rich blood. Your body's nourishment occurs at a faster pace. You shave off extra weight, your muscle tone is improved, your blood pressure goes down, you decrease your risk of heart disease, stress is reduced, your energy increases, and your mood improves. That's naming just a few of the benefits. All in addition to getting that healthy-looking glow! Here are a variety of aerobic activities that you may include in your 20- to 30-minute aerobic fitness activity: brisk walking (outdoors or on a treadmill), running (outdoors or on a treadmill), biking (stationary or outdoor), jogging in place, swimming, skating, rowing, hiking, jumping rope, race-walking, stair climbing, bench stepping, cross-country skiing (outdoor or skiing machine), using the elliptical trainer, engaging in low-impact aerobics and dancing.

Interval training is an aerobic fitness activity that alternates high-intensity activity levels with lower intensity effort. By challenging both your aerobic and anaerobic system at the same time, you're improving your body's ability to burn calories by leaps and bounds. You're building new muscle, which speeds up your metabolism of fat in general. You're getting an aerobic workout that burns plenty of calories! Your body will become a more efficient fat-burning machine.

Interval training is a great way to get around any fitness plateau you may have reached by doing the same fitness activity over and over again.

Strength Fitness

Strength fitness builds muscle. As you build muscle, you will lose fat. Muscles burn more calories than fat. When your body is at rest, strength fitness can actually speed up your metabolism! You can eat more healthful food without gaining weight or you can lose weight more quickly if you need to.

Strength training using weights can be done at a health club, a community or fitness center that has a weight room, with home equipment, or at a weight room in your apartment complex or community. You may use free weights (barbells and dumbbells), resistance-training machines (weights attached to cables and pulleys), or your own body weight (calisthenics). The benefit of going to a health club or center is that they provide professional training on the proper exercise form, which helps prevent injuries and which you can use both at the club and on your home equipment. Knowing the proper techniques can help you get the most out of your strength training.

Push-ups, crunches, lunges, and squats are also strengthening exercises. You only need to do strength fitness two or three times a week, and you need to rest at least a day in between to allow time for your muscles to heal, recover, and strengthen between workouts. It is a good idea to alternate your aerobic fitness with strength fitness. Swimming, cycling, and skiing are activities that improve both muscle strength and aerobic fitness.

Overall Fitness Program

To achieve fitness, most experts recommend either of the following:

- Moderate activity for 30 minutes a day, 5 days a week or more. Moderate activity is activity equal to a brisk walk.

- Vigorous exercise for 20 minutes a day, 3 times a week or more. Vigorous activity is activity that provides 70 percent or more of your maximum heart rate. The heart rate is how many times your heart beats in a minute. The maximum heart rate is the fastest the heart can beat at your maximum activity level. The maximum heart rate changes as you age. A percentage of the maximum heart rate is often used to determine the intensity of exercise.

  An easier way to determine if your heart rate is above 70 percent of your maximum heart rate is perceived exertion. This is a subjective measure of how hard you're working based primarily on your breathing. The scale goes from zero to ten, with level zero being how it feels to be at rest and level ten being an exertion so difficult you could probably only maintain it for a few seconds. Being at 70 percent of your maximum heart rate is about a level seven or eight. At level seven, you feel fatigue but are certain that you can maintain the pace for the rest of your session. Your breathing is deep, but you can still carry on a conversation. Level eight is slightly more vigorous; you may be able to still carry on a conversation, but you wouldn't want to.

Alternate your aerobic fitness or interval training with strength fitness during the week. You should plan on taking one day off for rest. Wear comfortable clothing, such as loose-fitting shorts or elasticized-waist knit lounge pants, a T-shirt, and athletic shoes. If you walk during your lunch hour at your workplace, you may just want to wear your normal work clothing; just make sure you are comfortable in it, and wear comfortable shoes.

Remember to start your aerobic and strength fitness program with flexibility exercises. Then, complete your aerobic and strength fitness with flexibility exercises to cool down your muscles and help prevent aches and pains.

Aerobic Fitness Day: Burn Fat/Cardiovascular Health
Flexibility Fitness: 5 minutes
Aerobic Fitness or Interval Training: 20–30 minutes
Flexibility Fitness: 5 minutes

Strength Fitness Day: Build Muscle/Tone Body
Flexibility Fitness: 5 minutes
Strength Fitness: 20–30 minutes
Flexibility Fitness: 5 minutes

Easy Aerobic Fitness, Walk More!

You can easily add aerobic fitness into your daily routine just by adding walking or walking more. Here are a few ways:

- Park your car in a parking spot at the far end of the lot, whether it's near work, the supermarket, the mall, or the cinema.
- If you take public transportation (bus, cab, subway, streetcar), get off ten blocks before your destination and walk the remainder of the way.
- Sign up for a weekly charity walk.
- Volunteer to walk dogs at an animal shelter or walk your own dog daily.
- In rainy or snowy weather, walk briskly around a mall for 20 or more minutes.
- Take the stairs instead of the elevator.
- Walk around the block several times while you wait for your child to take a music lesson.
- Walk around medical buildings if you have a long wait for a doctor's appointment. Ask the receptionist to give you an idea of how long your wait will be.

- If you dine out at lunch, walk to a nearby restaurant.
- If you have a meeting in another nearby building, leave 5 or 10 minutes early and walk to the building. Walk back to your building after the meeting.
- Walk to work, if you live near by.
- Walk to your shopping center if it is near where you live or work.

Interval Training

The key to burning fat is using interval workouts that alternate high-intensity levels with lower intensity effort. This type of workout simulates the start-and-stop motions with periods of sprinting to light jogging or rest, just like in sports. The great thing about interval workouts is that your body keeps burning calories long after the workout is over! You can use interval workouts in running, cycling, or swimming. Start with 20-minute workouts and increase the length of time as your endurance and strength builds.

Standard 20-minute Interval Workout

- 3 to 5 minutes of low intensity activity, such as a light jog, slow cycling, or slow swimming, to warm up
- 1 minute of moderate or high intensity activity, such as fast or very fast jogging, cycling, or swimming, followed by 1 minute of low intensity. Repeat this activity 6 to 8 times
- 3 to 5 minutes of low intensity activity, such as a light jog, slow cycling, or slow swimming, to slow down

Pinnacle 20-minute Interval Workout

Builds to a peak of high intensity activity alternating longer periods of high intensity activity with a steady period of low intensity activity and then coming back down

- 3 to 5 minutes of low intensity activity, such as a light jog, slow cycling, or slow swimming, to warm up
- 30 seconds of high intensity activity, such as very fast jogging, cycling, or swimming

- 1 minute of low intensity activity
- 45 seconds of high intensity activity
- 1 minute of low intensity activity
- 60 seconds of high intensity activity
- 1 minute of low intensity activity
- 90 seconds of high intensity activity
- 1 minute of low intensity activity
- 60 seconds of high intensity activity
- 1 minute of low intensity activity
- 45 seconds of high intensity activity
- 1 minute of low intensity activity
- 30 seconds of high intensity activity
- 3 to 5 minutes of low intensity activity, such as a light jog, slow cycling, or slow swimming, to cool down

Flexibility Fitness Activity

Flexibility fitness should be performed before and after aerobic fitness or strength fitness during the week. Plan on doing some type of fitness activity five to six times a week. Keep in mind to go slowly and gently with deliberate movements, no bouncing; this is the key to creating and maintaining flexibility in your body.

Select a few of the exercises from the following list to add into your flexibility fitness workout.

Sun Salutation: The yoga series of movements known as the 'Sun Salutation' is great for limbering up the whole body in preparation for any flexibility, aerobic, or strengthening movement. It is a graceful sequence of 12 positions performed in one continuous exercise. Each position counteracts the one before, stretching the body in a different way and alternately expanding and contracting the chest to regulate the breathing. Start by practicing 4 rounds and gradually build up to 12 rounds.

- Stand erect with feet together and palms in the prayer position in front of your chest. Exhale.

- Continue inhaling as you raise your arms in a wide circle out to the sides and overhead. Stretch your arms back as you lift them to allow the fullest expansion of your chest. Press your palms together above your head and look up at your hands. Stretch up and hold your breath. Hold the position for a few seconds with body in pose, breath held, eyes focused, and mind silent.

- Breathe out as you bend forward from the waist, keeping palms together, tucking your head, and keeping your back straight as long as you can. When you've bent as far forward as you can comfortably, grasp the back of your ankles, calves, or thighs, bend your elbows, pull your upper body gently toward your legs, and tuck your chin toward your chest. Hold your breath out. Hold the position for a few seconds with body in pose, breath held, eyes focused, and mind silent.

- Breathe in as you release your legs and stand up. Breathing out, immediately lunge forward with your right leg, keeping your toes tucked under. Support weight on both hands, right foot, left knee, and toes of the left foot. Tilt the head back; look up. Inhale and retain breath.

- Bring your right foot back next to your left foot. Straighten your body into a "plank" position.

- Hold your breath out as you lower your body so that your chin, chest, and knees touch the floor (toes are still tucked under). When your knees touch the floor, relax the held breath and start to breathe.

- Continue breathing in as you curl your head back. Lift your chest and stomach. Keep your hipbones on the floor, point your toes and bend back. Look up and back. Hold your breath. Hold the position for a few seconds with body in pose, breath held, eyes focused, and mind silent.

- Breathe out as you push your hips up and heels down into an inverted "V" position. Tuck your chin to your chest. Hold your breath out. Hold the position for a few seconds with body in pose, breath held, eyes focused, and mind silent.

- Start to breathe in as you bring your left foot forward between your hands and lunge forward with your left leg. Continue breathing in as you raise your arms in a wide circle to the sides and overhead, with palms together, looking up at your hands. Hold your breath. Hold the position for a few seconds with body in pose, breath held, eyes focused, and mind silent. Note: Alternate the leg you lunge forward with in this step as you did in previous steps to keep your right knee off the floor if you can.

- Breathe out as you bring your right foot forward next to the left. Grasp the back of your ankles, calves, or thighs. Bend your elbows. Pull your upper body gently toward your legs, and tuck your chin toward your chest. Hold your breath out. Hold the position for a few seconds with body in pose, breath held, eyes focused, and mind silent.

- Breathe in as you straighten, bringing your arms in a wide circle out to the sides and overhead, palms together. Look up at your hands and stretch. Hold your breath.

- Breathe out as you bring your arms in a circle down to the sides and back to your chest with palms together as in the first step.

Pelvic Tilt: Lie on your back with knees bent and arms at your side. Tighten stomach muscles and flatten the small of your back against the floor, without pushing down on the legs. Hold the tilt for five seconds, and then slowly relax. Repeat ten times.

Single Knee to Chest: Lie on your back with knees bent. Perform a pelvic tilt; then grasp your right knee with your hands, and gently pull your knee toward your chest. Hold for a count of 10. Return to starting position. Repeat with left leg. Do two times for each leg.

Double Knee to Chest: Lie on your back with knees bent. Perform a pelvic tilt; then grasp both knees with your hands, and gently pull toward your chest. Hold for a count of 10. Return to starting position. Do two times.

Back Rotation: Lie on your back with your right knee bent. Grasp your right knee with your left hand and gently pull to the left side until you feel a stretch. Keep your shoulders on the floor. Hold for a count of 10. Return to the starting position and repeat with your left knee. Do two times.

Hamstring Stretch: Lie on your back and grasp the back of the thigh of your right leg with both hands. Bend your hip up so your knee is facing the ceiling. Straighten your leg, raising your foot toward the ceiling. Your opposite leg should be flat against the floor. Hold for a count of 10. Return to the starting position and repeat with your left thigh. Do two times for each leg.

Heel Stretch: Lean against a wall and put your right foot forward. Keep your left foot flat and knee straight. Lower your body toward the wall by bending your elbows. Hold for a count of 10. Return to the starting position and repeat with your left leg forward and right leg stretched behind. Do two times for each leg.

Quadriceps Stretch: Brace yourself against a wall and grasp your right foot or ankle behind you. Gently pull it toward your buttocks, keeping your back straight—no arching. Hold for a count of 10. Return to the starting position and repeat with the left foot. Do two times for each leg.

Lunge: Take a large step forward with your right foot. Place your hands on your right knee and lean forward, bending your knee at a 90-degree angle, keeping your left knee in line with your left ankle. Hold for a count of 10. Return to the starting position and repeat with the left foot. Do two times for each leg.

Back Arm Stretch: With arms extended behind your back, interlace your fingers and push your arms up and back. Keep your chest out and head erect. Hold for a count of 10. Do two times.

Waist Stretch: Stand straight with your feet spread comfortably apart. Clasp your hands above your head and lean to the right from the waist. Straighten up and slowly bend to the left. Straighten up and slowly bend to the right. Bend from right to left, then left to right, two times.

Strengthening Fitness Activity

Strength fitness should be performed two to three times a week, alternating with your aerobic fitness day. Complete the strength fitness program with the flexibility fitness program to cool down your muscles and help prevent aches and pains.

When you lift weights, perform each movement slowly and deliberately. Specific weight-lifting movements are performed for a specific number of repetitions and a series of repetitions is called a set. Use 5-pound dumbbells and 2- to 3½-pound ankle weights to begin, progressing to 10-pound dumbbells, and 5-pound ankle weights as your strength improves. These weight sizes are not a rule, choose your level of weight depending on your current level of strength fitness; you may want to start out with 2-pound dumbbells and 1- to 1½-pound ankle weights and progress to 3- to 5-pound dumbbells and 2½- to 5-pound ankle weights. The key is to start with a low weight and progress to heavier weights as your strength builds.

Select a few of the exercises from the following list to add into your strengthening fitness workout.

Biceps Curl: Stand straight with arms at your sides, holding a dumbbell in each hand. Bend your arms and slowly raise the dumbbell toward your shoulders. Return to the starting position by lowering the weights slowly to your sides. Do two to three sets of 8 repetitions, resting about thirty seconds between sets.

Overhead Press: Stand with your feet shoulder-width apart, holding a dumbbell in each hand. Keep your back straight and raise your hands to your shoulder. Then raise both your arms toward the ceiling, so that the weights are above your head and the end of each weight is touching the other. Return to starting position by lowering the weights slowly to shoulder level. Do two to three sets of 8 repetitions, resting about thirty seconds between sets.

French Press: Stand straight and grasp a dumbbell at one end with both hands. Lift the weight overhead, fully extending both arms. Lower the weight slowly behind your head as far as you can, keeping your elbows pointed upward. Then, return to the starting position by slowly raising the weight so your arms are fully extended. Do two to three sets of 8 repetitions, resting about thirty seconds between sets.

Lateral Raise: Stand with your feet shoulder-width apart, holding a dumbbell in each hand, with your arms at your sides. Gently raise your arms out to the sides until your elbows are slightly higher than your shoulders. Lower your arms to the starting position. Do two to three sets of 8 repetitions, resting about thirty seconds between sets.

Arm Row: Stand in front of a chair and hold a weight in your left hand. Bending at your hips, lean forward and balance yourself on the chair with your right hand. Lift the weight to your side, and gently pull your left arm up, bending your elbow, to your chest. Then bend your elbow up behind you. Return to the starting position by slowly lowering the weight. Do two to three sets of 8 repetitions, resting about thirty seconds between sets. Repeat with your right arm.

Triceps Kickback: Stand in front of a chair and hold a weight in your left hand. Bending at your hips, lean forward and balance yourself on the chair with your right hand. Lift the weight to your side, and then bend your elbow up behind you. Slowly swing your forearm back, straightening your elbow. The weight should be a just a bit above the level of your back. Return to the starting position by lowering the weight slowly. Do two to three sets of 8 repetitions, resting about thirty seconds between sets. Repeat with your right arm.

Butterfly Curl: Lie on your back on the floor, holding a dumbbell in each hand. Extend arms to hold the weights straight above your chest. Slowly swing your hands out and lower them to the floor. Return to starting position by slowly raising the weights to above your chest. Do two to three sets of 8 repetitions, resting about thirty seconds between sets.

Push-Up: Kneeling on the floor, lean forward and place your hands shoulder-width apart on the floor. Point your fingers inward and your elbows outward. In this upright position, your arms and back should be straight, with knees touching the floor. Slowly lower your chest to the floor, keeping your back straight. Push up slowly, straightening your arms. Return to the starting position by slowly pushing up, straightening your arms. Do two to three sets of 8 repetitions, resting about thirty seconds between sets. Repeat with your right arm.

Basic Crunch: Lie on your back, with your arms across your chest or hands behind your head. Keeping your lower back on the floor, contract your abdominals and lift your shoulders. Slowing crunch your ribcage towards your pelvis. Return to starting position. Do two to three sets of 8 repetitions, resting about thirty seconds between sets.

Squat: Stand with your feet shoulder-width apart and your toes pointed straight ahead. With your feet flat on the floor, lower yourself into the squat position (just like sitting in a chair), extending your arms straight ahead as you do, looking forward. Keep your knees and ankles aligned; your knees should not extend beyond the ankles. Return to the starting position by slowly rising to the standing position. Do two to three sets of 8 repetitions, resting about thirty seconds between sets.

Leg Curl: Put an ankle-weight on each ankle. Holding on to the back of a chair, slowly bend your right knee until it is approximately parallel to the floor. Return to the starting position by lowering your leg slowly to the floor. Do two to three sets of 8 repetitions, resting about thirty seconds between sets. Repeat with your left leg.

Leg Lifts: With an ankle-weight on each ankle and holding onto the back of a chair, slowly lift your right leg behind you. Without straining, bending your knee slightly. Return to the starting position by slowly lowering your leg to the floor. Do two to three sets of 8 repetitions, resting about thirty seconds between sets. Repeat with your left leg.

Leg Extension: With an ankle-weight on each ankle, sit in a chair and slowly raise your right foot until your knee is straight and your leg is approximately parallel to the floor. Hold for a count of 3. Return to the starting position by slowly lowering your leg to the floor. Do two to three sets of 8 repetitions, resting about thirty seconds between sets. Repeat with your left leg

Cross Ankle Lift: With an ankle-weight on each ankle, sit in a chair and stretch out your legs in front of you. Cross your legs at the ankle and hold for a count of three. Return to the starting position by slowly lowering your leg to the floor. Do two to three sets of 8 repetitions, resting about thirty seconds between sets.

Abdominal Core Specific Activity

Your abdominal core is supported by four paired muscles in the abdominal wall. They fill all the space between the ribcage and pelvis. These muscles are the transversus abdominis, external obliques, internal obliques, and rectus abdominis.

The transversus abdominis is the deepest of the four, consisting of horizontal muscle fibers, and surrounding the abdomen like a girdle. Contraction of these muscles, as in pulling in your stomach, reduces the diameter of the abdomen. An easy way to feel the action of the transversus is to wrap your hands around the sides of your abdomen and cough.

The external obliques are muscles attached to the ribs and extending diagonally down the sides of your waist. Tightening of both sides causes firming of the abdomen and assists in bending of the torso.

The internal obliques lie between the transversus and the external obliques, and also extend diagonally down the sides of your waist. Contraction of the internal obliques results in side bending or rotation of the spine and ribcage (trunk). Tightening of both sides causes firming of the abdomen and assists in bending of the torso. The oblique muscles work synergetically in the rotation of the trunk; rotating the trunk to the right involves simultaneous contraction of the right internal oblique and the left external oblique.

The rectus abdominis is the six-pack muscles that help your upper body bend and maintain good posture. These muscles mainly bend the trunk (used in crunch or roll-up), but also assists the other three abdominal muscles in firming the abdomen. If you lie on your back with your knees bent and lift your head, you are activating the rectus abdominis. If you inhale deeply at the same time, you also activate the transversus abdominis. And if you also twist your shoulders alternately left to right, you activate the obliques.

Select a few of the exercises from the following list to add into your abdominal core fitness workout, keeping these things in mind:

- Work your abdominals 2 or 3 days a week. These muscles grow when they are at rest, not when you are working them, so give them some time in-between workouts to grow and strengthen.

- Work your abdominals at the beginning of your overall fitness activity, not at the end when you may be more likely to take shortcuts just to finish up.

- When working your abdominals, go slow to maximize intensity. The slower you go, the higher the intensity. The higher the intensity, the stronger the abdominals.

- Vary your abdominal exercises during each workout session.

Roll-Up: Great all-around abdominal exercise. Lie on your back with your arms and legs extended, feet flexed. Inhale. Exhale as you reach your arms up and forward and roll your head toward your chest, lifting your head and shoulders off the floor. Press your inner thighs together and begin to pull your navel in toward your spine. Slowly peel off the floor until you are sitting in a letter "C" shape (back rounded, head toward knees, and arms extended). Slowly reverse the movement, inhaling and squeezing your abdominals as you roll back down to the floor. Repeat the sequence 6 to 10 times.

Crisscross: Works the obliques. Lie on your back with your knees above your hips, calves parallel to floor, and hands behind your head. Raise your head and shoulders, tightening your abdominals and twisting to the left as you extend your right leg. Hold for 3 seconds and then switch sides. Hold for another 3 seconds. This is one repetition. Repeat for 5 more repetitions, alternating legs.

Reverse Curl: Works the lower abdominals. Lie on your back and place your hands, palms down, alongside your thighs. Bend your hips and knees to form a 90-degree angle: thighs vertical and lower legs horizontal. Slowly contract your abdominal muscles, lifting your hips about 2 to 4 inches off the floor. Hold, and then slowly lower.

Seated Balance: Sit on the floor with your knees bent and feet flat. Extend your arms straight in front of you. Lift your feet so that they are parallel to the floor and balance on your sitting bones. Hold for three breaths. Do one time only.

Chest Raise: Great lower back strengthener! Lie on your stomach, keeping your hips and pelvis flat. With your hands under your chin or in a push-up position to help you in lifting, contract your lower back muscles and lift your chest about 30 degrees off the floor. Hold, and then slowly lower.

Crunch Combo: Works the upper abdominals and obliques. Lie on your back on a small rug on the floor, with your arms across your chest or hands behind your head. Keeping your lower back on the floor, contract your abdominals and lift your shoulders. Twist your body slightly to the left and lower yourself to the floor, and then crunch forward by lifting your shoulders with no twisting. Lower, then lift and twist toward the right. Lower body and crunch forward. Return to starting position. Do two to three sets of 8 repetitions, resting about thirty seconds between sets.

Weighted Crunch: Works the upper abdominals. Lie on your back with your knees bent. Hold a light dumbbell in each hand, and stretch your arms straight back behind you. Slowly crunch your rib cage toward your pelvis. Return to starting position. Do 12 to 15 repetitions.

Bicycle: Works the upper and lower abdominals. Lie on your back with your knees bent 90 degrees and your hands behind your ears. Pump your legs back and forth, bicycle-style, as you rotate your torso from side to side by moving an armpit (not your elbow) toward the opposite knee. Do 20 repetitions.

Pulse-Up: Works the lower abdominals. Lie with your hands underneath your tailbone and your legs raised and pointed straight up toward the ceiling, perpendicular to your torso. Pull your navel inward, and flex your glutes as you lift your hips a few inches off the floor. Lower your hips. Do 12 repetitions.

Seated Crunch: Works the lower abdominals and you can even do this at work! Sit up straight in a firm, armless chair. Grab the chair's edges just in front of your hips. While supporting yourself with your hands, slowly draw your knees up toward your chest while breathing out, keeping your lower back pressed against the chair. Hold and then slowly lower your knees. Do 12 repetitions.

Speed Rotation: Works the obliques. Stand while holding a dumbbell with both hands in front of your midsection. Twist 90 degrees to the right, then 180 degrees to your left. Keep your abdominals tight and move fast. Return to center. Alternate the side you start with. Do 10 repetitions each side.

Side Bend: Works the obliques. Hold a pair of lightweight dumbbells over your head, in line with your shoulders, with your elbows slightly bent. Keep your back straight, and slowly bend directly to your left side as far as possible without twisting your upper body. Pause and feel the stretch, return to an upright position, then bend to your right side as far as possible.

Bridge: Strengthen your transversus abdominis with this movement. Position yourself as if you are going to do a push-up, but bend your elbows and rest your weight on your forearms instead of your hands. Your body should form a straight line from your shoulders to your ankles. Pull your abdominals in (suck in your stomach) and hold for 20 seconds, breathing steadily. As you develop more endurance, increase the hold time for 60 seconds. Do 1 to 2 repetitions.

Superman Bridge: Strengthen your transversus abdominis with this movement. Position yourself as if you are going to do a push-up. Lift and stretch out your right arm and your left leg off the floor at the same time. Hold for 3 to 5 seconds. This is one repetition. Return to starting position, then repeat, lifting your left arm and right leg this time. Do 6 to 10 repetitions each side.

Chapter 4

Chart Your Fitness Progress

This chapter contains the worksheets for you to use to chart your fitness progress and activities during your 6-week *Transform Your Core* program. The charts and the number of each included are:

- One Fitness Progress Chart worksheet, with formulas to estimate your BMI and estimate your lean body weight, fat body weight, and body fat percentage based on your height, weight, waist, wrist, hip, and forearm measurements for each week.

- Six Fitness Activity Chart worksheets to record the type of fitness activity and amount of time spent performing it and the stress reduction technique practiced during each day of the week.

- Ten Strength Training Log worksheets to record your exercise weight loads and the number of repetitions for the strengthening fitness exercises described in Chapter 3.

- Eight Core Strength Training Log worksheets to record your exercise weight loads and the number of repetitions for the abdominal core strengthening fitness exercises described in Chapter 3.

- Seven Nutrition Log worksheets to record your daily meals and their calorie total with a breakdown of calories for the breakfast, lunch, dinner, and snack meals; as well as the calorie percentage of protein, fat, and carbohydrates in each of those meals

You may want to make additional photocopies of each worksheet for ongoing use after six weeks. For ease in writing in your entries, you may wish to enlarge each worksheet as you copy it.

Fitness Progress Chart

| Height (feet) | | | | | | | | | | |
| Height (inches) | | | | | | | | | | |

Date	Weight (pounds)	Chest (inches)	Waist (inches)	Hips (inches)	Wrist (inches)	Forearm (inches)	Estimated Lean Body Weight	Estimated Body Fat Weight	Estimated Body Fat Percentage	Estimated Body Mass Index (BMI)

Formulas to Calculate:

Estimated Body Mass Index (BMI): (Weight x 704.5) / ((Height in Feet x 12 + Height in Inches) / (Height in Feet x 12 + Height in Inches))

Estimated Lean Body Weight Formula For Women:

Factor 1	(Weight x 0.732) + 8.987
Factor 2	Wrist measurement (at fullest point) / 3.140
Factor 3	Waist measurement (at naval) x 0.157
Factor 4	Hip measurement (at fullest point) x 0.249
Factor 5	Forearm measurement (at fullest point) x 0.434
Estimated Lean Body Weight	Factor 1 + Factor 2 - Factor 3 - Factor 4 + Factor 5
Estimated Body Fat Weight	Weight - Lean Body Weight
Estimated Body Fat Percentage	(Body Fat Weight x 100) / Weight

Estimated Lean Body Weight Formula For Men:

Factor 1	(Weight x 1.082) + 94.42
Factor 2	Waist measurement x 4.15
Estimated Lean Body Weight	Factor 1 - Factor 2
Estimated Body Fat Weight	Weight - Lean Body Weight
Estimated Body Fat Percentage	(Body Fat Weight x 100) / Weight

Fitness Activity Chart

Week of:

Day	Flexibility	Time	Aerobic	Time	Strength	Time	Stress Reduction Technique
Monday							
Tuesday							
Wednesday							
Thursday							
Friday							
Saturday							
Sunday							

Fitness Activity Chart

Week of:

Day	Flexibility	Time	Aerobic	Time	Strength	Time	Stress Reduction Technique
Monday							
Tuesday							
Wednesday							
Thursday							
Friday							
Saturday							
Sunday							

Fitness Activity Chart

Week of:

Day	Flexibility	Time	Aerobic	Time	Strength	Time	Stress Reduction Technique
Monday							
Tuesday							
Wednesday							
Thursday							
Friday							
Saturday							
Sunday							

Fitness Activity Chart

Week of:

Day	Flexibility	Time	Aerobic	Time	Strength	Time	Stress Reduction Technique
Monday							
Tuesday							
Wednesday							
Thursday							
Friday							
Saturday							
Sunday							

Fitness Activity Chart

Week of:

Day	Flexibility	Time	Aerobic	Time	Strength	Time	Stress Reduction Technique
Monday							
Tuesday							
Wednesday							
Thursday							
Friday							
Saturday							
Sunday							

Fitness Activity Chart

Week of:

Day	Flexibility	Time	Aerobic	Time	Strength	Time	Stress Reduction Technique
Monday							
Tuesday							
Wednesday							
Thursday							
Friday							
Saturday							
Sunday							

Strength Training Log

Date:
Workout Duration:

	Exercise	Set 1	Set 2	Set 3	Set 4	Set 5	Set 6
UPPER BODY	Biceps Curl	—	—	—	—	—	—
	Overhead Press	—	—	—	—	—	—
	French Press	—	—	—	—	—	—
	Lateral Raise	—	—	—	—	—	—
	Arm Row	—	—	—	—	—	—
	Triceps Kickback	—	—	—	—	—	—
	Butterfly Curl	—	—	—	—	—	—
	Push-Up	—	—	—	—	—	—
LEGS	Squat	—	—	—	—	—	—
	Leg Curl	—	—	—	—	—	—
	Leg Lifts	—	—	—	—	—	—
	Leg Extension	—	—	—	—	—	—
	Cross Ankle Lift	—	—	—	—	—	—
AB	Basic Crunch	—	—	—	—	—	—

Note: Per set, per relevant exercise, record the amount of weight lifted and then, after the " | ", record the number of repetitions you complete.

Strength Training Log

Date:
Workout Duration:

	Exercise	Set 1	Set 2	Set 3	Set 4	Set 5	Set 6
UPPER BODY	Biceps Curl	—	—	—	—	—	—
	Overhead Press	—	—	—	—	—	—
	French Press	—	—	—	—	—	—
	Lateral Raise	—	—	—	—	—	—
	Arm Row	—	—	—	—	—	—
	Triceps Kickback	—	—	—	—	—	—
	Butterfly Curl	—	—	—	—	—	—
	Push-Up	—	—	—	—	—	—
LEGS	Squat	—	—	—	—	—	—
	Leg Curl	—	—	—	—	—	—
	Leg Lifts	—	—	—	—	—	—
	Leg Extension	—	—	—	—	—	—
	Cross Ankle Lift	—	—	—	—	—	—
AB	Basic Crunch	—	—	—	—	—	—

Note: Per set, per relevant exercise, record the amount of weight lifted and then, after the " | ", record the number of repetitions you complete.

Strength Training Log

Date:
Workout Duration:

	Exercise	Set 1	Set 2	Set 3	Set 4	Set 5	Set 6
UPPER BODY	Biceps Curl	—	—	—	—	—	—
	Overhead Press	—	—	—	—	—	—
	French Press	—	—	—	—	—	—
	Lateral Raise	—	—	—	—	—	—
	Arm Row	—	—	—	—	—	—
	Triceps Kickback	—	—	—	—	—	—
	Butterfly Curl	—	—	—	—	—	—
	Push-Up	—	—	—	—	—	—
LEGS	Squat	—	—	—	—	—	—
	Leg Curl	—	—	—	—	—	—
	Leg Lifts	—	—	—	—	—	—
	Leg Extension	—	—	—	—	—	—
	Cross Ankle Lift	—	—	—	—	—	—
AB	Basic Crunch						

Note: Per set, per relevant exercise, record the amount of weight lifted and then, after the " | ", record the number of repetitions you complete.

Strength Training Log

Date:
Workout Duration:

	Exercise	Set 1	Set 2	Set 3	Set 4	Set 5	Set 6
BODY	Biceps Curl	—	—	—	—	—	—
	Overhead Press	—	—	—	—	—	—
UPPER	French Press	—	—	—	—	—	—
	Lateral Raise	—	—	—	—	—	—
	Arm Row	—	—	—	—	—	—
	Triceps Kickback	—	—	—	—	—	—
	Butterfly Curl	—	—	—	—	—	—
	Push-Up						
LEGS	Squat						
	Leg Curl	—	—	—	—	—	—
	Leg Lifts	—	—	—	—	—	—
	Leg Extension	—	—	—	—	—	—
	Cross Ankle Lift	—	—	—	—	—	—
AB	Basic Crunch	—	—	—	—	—	—

Note: Per set, per relevant exercise, record the amount of weight lifted and then, after the " | ", record the number of repetitions you complete.

Strength Training Log

Date:
Workout Duration:

	Exercise	Set 1	Set 2	Set 3	Set 4	Set 5	Set 6
UPPER BODY	Biceps Curl	—	—	—	—	—	—
	Overhead Press	—	—	—	—	—	—
	French Press	—	—	—	—	—	—
	Lateral Raise	—	—	—	—	—	—
	Arm Row	—	—	—	—	—	—
	Triceps Kickback	—	—	—	—	—	—
	Butterfly Curl	—	—	—	—	—	—
	Push-Up	—	—	—	—	—	—
LEGS	Squat	—	—	—	—	—	—
	Leg Curl	—	—	—	—	—	—
	Leg Lifts	—	—	—	—	—	—
	Leg Extension	—	—	—	—	—	—
	Cross Ankle Lift	—	—	—	—	—	—
AB	Basic Crunch	—	—	—	—	—	—

Note: Per set, per relevant exercise, record the amount of weight lifted and then, after the "|", record the number of repetitions you complete.

Strength Training Log

Date:
Workout Duration:

	Exercise	Set 1	Set 2	Set 3	Set 4	Set 5	Set 6
UPPER BODY	Biceps Curl	—	—	—	—	—	—
	Overhead Press	—	—	—	—	—	—
	French Press	—	—	—	—	—	—
	Lateral Raise	—	—	—	—	—	—
	Arm Row	—	—	—	—	—	—
	Triceps Kickback	—	—	—	—	—	—
	Butterfly Curl	—	—	—	—	—	—
	Push-Up	—	—	—	—	—	—
LEGS	Squat	—	—	—	—	—	—
	Leg Curl	—	—	—	—	—	—
	Leg Lifts	—	—	—	—	—	—
	Leg Extension	—	—	—	—	—	—
	Cross Ankle Lift	—	—	—	—	—	—
AB	Basic Crunch	—	—	—	—	—	—

Note: Per set, per relevant exercise, record the amount of weight lifted and then, after the " | ", record the number of repetitions you complete.

Strength Training Log

Date:
Workout Duration:

	Exercise	Set 1	Set 2	Set 3	Set 4	Set 5	Set 6
UPPER BODY	Biceps Curl	—	—	—	—	—	—
	Overhead Press	—	—	—	—	—	—
	French Press	—	—	—	—	—	—
	Lateral Raise	—	—	—	—	—	—
	Arm Row	—	—	—	—	—	—
	Triceps Kickback	—	—	—	—	—	—
	Butterfly Curl	—	—		—	—	—
	Push-Up	—	—		—	—	—
LEGS	Squat	—	—	—	—	—	—
	Leg Curl	—	—	—	—	—	—
	Leg Lifts	—	—	—	—	—	—
	Leg Extension	—	—	—	—	—	—
	Cross Ankle Lift	—	—	—	—	—	—
AB	Basic Crunch						

Note: Per set, per relevant exercise, record the amount of weight lifted and then, after the " | ", record the number of repetitions you complete.

Strength Training Log

Date:
Workout Duration:

	Exercise	Set 1	Set 2	Set 3	Set 4	Set 5	Set 6
UPPER BODY	Biceps Curl	—	—	—	—	—	—
	Overhead Press	—	—	—	—	—	—
	French Press	—	—	—	—	—	—
	Lateral Raise	—	—	—	—	—	—
	Arm Row	—	—	—	—	—	—
	Triceps Kickback	—	—	—	—	—	—
	Butterfly Curl	—	—	—	—	—	—
	Push-Up	—	—	—	—	—	—
LEGS	Squat	—	—	—	—	—	—
	Leg Curl	—	—	—	—	—	—
	Leg Lifts	—	—	—	—	—	—
	Leg Extension	—	—	—	—	—	—
	Cross Ankle Lift	—	—	—	—	—	—
AB	Basic Crunch	—	—	—	—	—	—

Note: Per set, per relevant exercise, record the amount of weight lifted and then, after the " | ", record the number of repetitions you complete.

Strength Training Log

Date:
Workout Duration:

	Exercise	Set 1	Set 2	Set 3	Set 4	Set 5	Set 6
UPPER BODY	Biceps Curl	—	—	—	—	—	—
	Overhead Press	—	—	—	—	—	—
	French Press	—	—	—	—	—	—
	Lateral Raise	—	—	—	—	—	—
	Arm Row	—	—	—	—	—	—
	Triceps Kickback	—	—	—	—	—	—
	Butterfly Curl	—	—	—	—	—	—
	Push-Up	—	—	—	—	—	—
LEGS	Squat	—	—	—	—	—	—
	Leg Curl	—	—	—	—	—	—
	Leg Lifts	—	—	—	—	—	—
	Leg Extension	—	—	—	—	—	—
	Cross Ankle Lift	—	—	—	—	—	—
AB	Basic Crunch	—	—	—	—	—	—

Note: Per set, per relevant exercise, record the amount of weight lifted and then, after the " | ", record the number of repetitions you complete.

Strength Training Log

Date:
Workout Duration:

	Exercise	Set 1	Set 2	Set 3	Set 4	Set 5	Set 6
UPPER BODY	Biceps Curl	—	—	—	—	—	—
	Overhead Press	—	—	—	—	—	—
	French Press	—	—	—	—	—	—
	Lateral Raise	—	—	—	—	—	—
	Arm Row	—	—	—	—	—	—
	Triceps Kickback	—	—	—	—	—	—
	Butterfly Curl	—	—	—	—	—	—
	Push-Up	—	—	—	—	—	—
LEGS	Squat	—	—	—	—	—	—
	Leg Curl	—	—	—	—	—	—
	Leg Lifts	—	—	—	—	—	—
	Leg Extension	—	—	—	—	—	—
	Cross Ankle Lift	—	—	—	—	—	—
AB	Basic Crunch	—	—	—	—	—	—

Note: Per set, per relevant exercise, record the amount of weight lifted and then, after the " | ", record the number of repetitions you complete.

Core Strength Training Log

Date:
Workout Duration:

	Exercise	Set 1	Set 2	Set 3	Set 4	Set 5	Set 6
CORE	Roll-Up	—	—	—	—	—	—
	Crisscross	—	—	—	—	—	—
	Reverse Curl	—	—	—	—	—	—
	Seated Balance	—	—	—	—	—	—
	Chest Raise	—	—	—	—	—	—
	Crunch Combo	—	—	—	—	—	—
	Weighted Crunch	—	—	—	—	—	—
ABS	Bicycle	—	—	—	—	—	—
	Pulse-Up	—	—	—	—	—	—
	Seated Crunch	—	—	—	—	—	—
	Speed Rotation	—	—	—	—	—	—
	Side Bend	—	—	—	—	—	—
	Bridge	—	—	—	—	—	—
	Superman Bridge	—	—	—	—	—	—

Note: Per set, per relevant exercise, record the number of repetitions you complete.

Core Strength Training Log

Date:
Workout Duration:

Exercise		Set 1	Set 2	Set 3	Set 4	Set 5	Set 6
ABS	Roll-Up	—	—	—	—	—	—
	Crisscross	—	—	—	—	—	—
	Reverse Curl	—	—	—	—	—	—
	Seated Balance	—	—	—	—	—	—
	Chest Raise	—	—	—	—	—	—
	Crunch Combo	—	—	—	—	—	—
	Weighted Crunch	—	—	—	—	—	—
CORE	Bicycle	—	—	—	—	—	—
	Pulse-Up	—	—	—	—	—	—
	Seated Crunch	—	—	—	—	—	—
	Speed Rotation	—	—	—	—	—	—
	Side Bend	—	—	—	—	—	—
	Bridge	—	—	—	—	—	—
	Superman Bridge	—	—	—	—	—	—

Note: Per set, per relevant exercise, record the number of repetitions you complete.

Core Strength Training Log

Date:
Workout Duration:

Exercise		Set 1	Set 2	Set 3	Set 4	Set 5	Set 6
Roll-Up	CORE	—	—	—	—	—	—
Crisscross	CORE	—	—	—	—	—	—
Reverse Curl	CORE			—			—
Seated Balance	CORE	—	—	—	—	—	—
Chest Raise	CORE	—	—	—	—	—	—
Crunch Combo	CORE	—	—	—	—	—	—
Weighted Crunch	ABS	—	—	—	—	—	—
Bicycle	ABS	—	—	—	—	—	—
Pulse-Up	ABS	—	—	—	—	—	—
Seated Crunch	ABS	—	—	—	—	—	—
Speed Rotation	ABS	—	—	—	—	—	—
Side Bend	ABS						
Bridge	ABS	—	—	—	—	—	—
Superman Bridge	ABS	—	—	—	—	—	—

Note: Per set, per relevant exercise, record the number of repetitions you complete.

Core Strength Training Log

Date:
Workout Duration:

Exercise		Set 1	Set 2	Set 3	Set 4	Set 5	Set 6
ABS	Roll-Up	—	—	—	—	—	—
	Crisscross	—	—	—	—	—	—
	Reverse Curl	—	—	—	—	—	—
	Seated Balance	—	—	—	—	—	—
	Chest Raise	—	—	—	—	—	—
	Crunch Combo	—	—	—	—	—	—
	Weighted Crunch	—	—	—	—	—	—
	Bicycle	—	—	—	—	—	—
	Pulse-Up	—	—	—	—	—	—
	Seated Crunch	—	—	—	—	—	—
CORE	Speed Rotation	—	—	—	—	—	—
	Side Bend	—	—	—	—	—	—
	Bridge	—	—	—	—	—	—
	Superman Bridge	—	—	—	—	—	—

Note: Per set, per relevant exercise, record the number of repetitions you complete.

Core Strength Training Log

Date:
Workout Duration:

	Exercise	Set 1	Set 2	Set 3	Set 4	Set 5	Set 6
CORE	Roll-Up	—	—	—	—	—	—
	Crisscross	—	—	—	—	—	—
	Reverse Curl	—	—	—	—	—	—
	Seated Balance	—	—	—	—	—	—
	Chest Raise	—	—	—	—	—	—
	Crunch Combo	—	—	—	—	—	—
	Weighted Crunch	—	—	—	—	—	—
ABS	Bicycle	—	—	—	—	—	—
	Pulse-Up	—	—	—	—	—	—
	Seated Crunch	—	—	—	—	—	—
	Speed Rotation	—	—	—	—	—	—
	Side Bend	—	—	—	—	—	—
	Bridge	—	—	—	—	—	—
	Superman Bridge	—	—	—	—	—	—

Note: Per set, per relevant exercise, record the number of repetitions you complete.

Core Strength Training Log

Date:
Workout Duration:

	Exercise	Set 1	Set 2	Set 3	Set 4	Set 5	Set 6
ABS	Roll-Up	—	—	—	—	—	—
	Crisscross	—	—	—	—	—	—
	Reverse Curl	—	—	—	—	—	—
	Seated Balance	—	—	—	—	—	—
	Chest Raise	—	—	—	—	—	—
	Crunch Combo	—	—	—	—	—	—
	Weighted Crunch	—	—	—	—	—	—
CORE	Bicycle	—	—	—	—	—	—
	Pulse-Up	—	—	—	—	—	—
	Seated Crunch	—	—	—	—	—	—
	Speed Rotation	—	—	—	—	—	—
	Side Bend	—	—	—	—	—	—
	Bridge	—	—	—	—	—	—
	Superman Bridge	—	—	—	—	—	—

Note: Per set, per relevant exercise, record the number of repetitions you complete.

Core Strength Training Log

Date:
Workout Duration:

Exercise		Set 1	Set 2	Set 3	Set 4	Set 5	Set 6
Roll-Up	CORE	—	—	—	—	—	—
Crisscross		—	—	—	—	—	—
Reverse Curl		—	—	—	—	—	—
Seated Balance		—	—	—	—	—	—
Chest Raise		—	—	—	—	—	—
Crunch Combo		—	—	—	—	—	—
Weighted Crunch		—	—	—	—	—	—
Bicycle	ABS	—	—	—	—	—	—
Pulse-Up		—	—	—	—	—	—
Seated Crunch		—	—	—	—	—	—
Speed Rotation		—	—	—	—	—	—
Side Bend		—	—	—	—	—	—
Bridge		—	—	—	—	—	—
Superman Bridge		—	—	—	—	—	—

Note: Per set, per relevant exercise, record the number of repetitions you complete.

Core Strength Training Log

Date:
Workout Duration:

Exercise		Set 1	Set 2	Set 3	Set 4	Set 5	Set 6
Roll-Up	ABS	—	—	—	—	—	—
Crisscross	ABS	—	—	—	—	—	—
Reverse Curl	ABS	—	—	—	—	—	—
Seated Balance	ABS	—	—	—	—	—	—
Chest Raise	ABS	—	—	—	—	—	—
Crunch Combo	ABS	—	—	—	—	—	—
Weighted Crunch	ABS	—	—	—	—	—	—
Bicycle	ABS	—	—	—	—	—	—
Pulse-Up	ABS	—	—	—	—	—	—
Seated Crunch	CORE	—	—	—	—	—	—
Speed Rotation	CORE	—	—	—	—	—	—
Side Bend	CORE	—	—	—	—	—	—
Bridge	CORE	—	—	—	—	—	—
Superman Bridge	CORE	—	—	—	—	—	—

Note: Per set, per relevant exercise, record the number of repetitions you complete.

Nutrition Log

Date:

Note: Record your daily percentages of protein, fat, and carbohydrate calories and then, after the " | ", record the number of calories for each in your meal. For example, 30% protein and 300 protein calories (30 | 300).

	Calories	Protein % | Calories	Fat % | Calories	Carbohydrate % | Calories
Breakfast Meal				
Lunch Meal				
Dinner Meal				
Snacks				
Daily Calorie Total	Total Calories	Protein Calories	Fat Calories	Carbohydrate Calories

Nutrition Log

Note: Record your daily percentages of protein, fat, and carbohydrate calories and then, after the " | ", record the number of calories for each in your meal. For example, 30% protein and 300 protein calories (30 | 300).

Date:

	Calories	Protein %	Calories	Fat %	Calories	Carbohydrate %	Calories
Breakfast Meal							
Lunch Meal							
Dinner Meal							
Snacks							
Daily Calorie Total	Total Calories	Protein Calories		Fat Calories		Carbohydrate Calories	

Nutrition Log

Note: Record your daily percentages of protein, fat, and carbohydrate calories and then, after the " | ", record the number of calories for each in your meal. For example, 30% protein and 300 protein calories (30 | 300).

Date:

	Calories	Protein %	Calories	Fat %	Calories	Carbohydrate %	Calories
Breakfast Meal							
Lunch Meal							
Dinner Meal							
Snacks							
Daily Calorie Total	Total Calories	Protein Calories		Fat Calories		Carbohydrate Calories	

Nutrition Log

Date:

Note: Record your daily percentages of protein, fat, and carbohydrate calories and then, after the " | ", record the number of calories for each in your meal. For example, 30% protein and 300 protein calories (30 | 300).

	Calories	Protein %	Protein Calories	Fat %	Fat Calories	Carbohydrate %	Carbohydrate Calories
Breakfast Meal							
Lunch Meal							
Dinner Meal							
Snacks							
Daily Calorie Total	Total Calories		Protein Calories		Fat Calories		Carbohydrate Calories

Nutrition Log

Date:

Note: Record your daily percentages of protein, fat, and carbohydrate calories and then, after the " | ", record the number of calories for each in your meal. For example, 30% protein and 300 protein calories (30 | 300).

	Calories	Protein %	Calories	Fat %	Calories	Carbohydrate %	Calories
Breakfast Meal							
Lunch Meal							
Dinner Meal							
Snacks							
Daily Calorie Total	Total Calories	Protein Calories		Fat Calories		Carbohydrate Calories	

Nutrition Log

Date:

Note: Record your daily percentages of protein, fat, and carbohydrate calories and then, after the "|", record the number of calories for each in your meal. For example, 30% protein and 300 protein calories (30 | 300).

	Calories	Protein %	Calories	Fat %	Calories	Carbohydrate %	Calories
Breakfast Meal							
Lunch Meal							
Dinner Meal							
Snacks							

	Total Calories	Protein Calories	Fat Calories	Carbohydrate Calories
Daily Calorie Total				

Nutrition Log

Date:

Note: Record your daily percentages of protein, fat, and carbohydrate calories and then, after the " | ", record the number of calories for each in your meal. For example, 30% protein and 300 protein calories (30 | 300).

	Calories	Protein %	Calories	Fat %	Calories	Carbohydrate %	Calories
Breakfast Meal							
Lunch Meal							
Dinner Meal							
Snacks							

	Total Calories	Protein Calories	Fat Calories	Carbohydrate Calories
Daily Calorie Total				

About the Author

In her previous books, *Building a Healthy Lifestyle: A Simple Nutrition and Fitness Approach*; *Easy and Healthful Mediterranean Cooking, Flavoring with Culinary Herbs: Tips, Recipes, and Cultivation*; and *The Essence of Herbal and Floral Teas*, Mary El-Baz presented an invaluable nutritional program for anyone to build a healthy lifestyle; a collection of savory, nutritious Mediterranean recipes; a guide on using culinary herbs to enhance the flavor, aroma, and appeal of foods; and a recipe guide on herbs and edible flowers to use in aromatic and healthful herbal and floral teas, tisanes, beverages, and desserts.

She now brings you *Transform Your Core 6-Week Workbook*, a simple diet, stress reduction, and fitness plan designed to help readers recognize what factors favor midsection weight gain, how to create and follow an eating plan that encourages weight loss, and which fitness activities to undertake to promote weight loss and target the firming and redefinition of their body core, the abdominal muscles.

Dr. El-Baz holds a doctorate in Holistic Nutrition and from Clayton College of Natural Health and degrees from the University of Missouri. She is currently completing her Doctor of Naturopathy degree from Clayton College.

Index

978-0-595-41697-4
0-595-41697-7